The Healing Power of Pets

The Healing Power of Pets

Harnessing the Amazing Ability of Pets to Make and Keep People Happy and Healthy

Dr. Marty Becker

with Danelle Morton

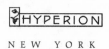

NEW YORK

Copyright © 2002 Dr. Marty Becker

LIBRARY OF CONGRESS CATALOGING-IN-PUBLICATION DATA

Becker, Marty
    The healing power of pets : harnessing the amazing ability of pets to make and keep people happy and healthy / Marty Becker, with Danelle Morton—1st ed.
        p. cm.
    Includes bibliographical references.
    ISBN 0-7868-6808-2
    1. Pets—Therapeutic use. I. Morton, Danelle. II. Title.
RM931.A65 B436 2002
615.8'515—dc21

                                                    2001039779

FIRST EDITION

10 9 8 7 6 5 4 3 2 1

WE DEDICATE THIS BOOK TO every pet companion who lavishes healing gifts on a human family. We owe you a great debt.

To the families who make sure their pets' health, happiness, and longevity is a priority.

To all health care providers who celebrate, protect, and nurture the integrative medicine concept of mind, body, and meaning and who use the healing power of pets to improve human health and well-being.

To the researchers who are finally proving what we've all believed to be true: that pets don't just make us feel good but are good for us.

To God for the gift of animals and the promise of another Garden of Eden in heaven.

Contents

Part One 21
The Healing Power of Pets

Part Two 183
The Pet Prescription

Part Three 225
Deepening the Bond

Acknowledgments

INTIMACY WITH A BELOVED PET or special animal makes millions of people feel as though they win the lottery every day. Unlike most things in life, with pets we comparatively give so little and are guaranteed of getting so much back in return.

I'd studied the healing power of pets for many years, had witnessed and been told hundreds of stories of medical miracles, and had even experienced the power of the Bond during my own illness. Even after having the idea for this book rattling around in my head for almost ten years, I had no way of knowing its thesis would be so widely accepted when we started our work. What a delight to have too much to cover rather than too little.

Starting out, I was confident I had enough stories, studies, and experience to write a good book. But thanks to my coauthor Danelle Morton's investigative reporting experience, talent for interviewing, and experience with writing books, we have what we hope you'll find is a great book. I thank Danelle not only for her partnership and teaching me the ropes of reporting and writing, but for the gift of her friendship.

I also want to thank the following people who helped with the researching, reviewing, or writing of significant portions of this book: Arden Moore, Anne Sellaro, Rolan and Susan Tripp, and Sandra Wendel. You gave a 110 percent to this team effort and we're very grateful. We're also very grateful to Stephanie Voss, Bill Krauss, and Roland Riksheim for their support and help with crisis management during the hectic journey of producing this book.

I want to express my deep appreciation for the more than 350 of my veterinary colleagues, physicians, and other health care providers, researchers, academicians, writers, patients, and pet lovers who allowed us to interview them for this book. Although we weren't able to feature all of your information or stories, you're part of the recipe. I would like to single out for special recognition some Bond fanatics and incredible supporters: R. K. Anderson, Scott Campbell, Steve Garner, John Payne, Jack Stephens, Chuck Wayner, and Jim Wilson.

Thanks to our peerless agent and friend David Vigliano, who can speak loudly and carries a big stick. We're in awe of your knowledge of every aspect of writing.

All the folks at our publisher Hyperion deserve a thank you but especially two people. To our talented editor, Leslie Wells, whose steadfast guidance, consistent enthusiasm, and firm sense for what we needed to say and what we could do without kept us working hard without losing our optimism and joy. Special gratitude is in order for Carrie Covert, who on more than one occasion seemed less like an editorial assistant and more like a magician in solving problems, moving mountains, and granting wishes.

We couldn't have done this book without our beloved families, whose love gave us the "inspiration for the perspiration" and in whose loving arms we cradled ourselves at the end of twelve- to eighteen-hour days.

Finally, to my pets and animals, who graced me with their gifts of love, loyalty, and laughter and who allowed me to test my assignments and theories of deepening the Bond on them.

The Healing Power of Pets

Preface

The Bond
The Cementing of Science and Soul

I'M THE KIND OF PERSON who bolts out of bed in the morning with his mind already running through the day and weeks ahead. Yet on a Wednesday morning in November of 2000, my body wouldn't cooperate. I leapt from bed as usual, but when my feet hit the ground, they were as numb as if I'd just sleepwalked barefoot through a knee-deep field of snow. When I reached out to steady myself on the bed, I discovered the same lack of sensation from my fingertips to my elbow. Maybe I'd just slept wrong, I tried to convince myself as I pounded to the bathroom on wooden feet.

I flexed my fingers and arms trying to pump feeling into my limbs as I looked myself in the eye in the bathroom mirror. All the while, my doctor self ran through the many major medical problems these symptoms could point to. I was so scared. My older brother Bob had awoken with these same symptoms just three years earlier, and was subsequently diagnosed with multiple sclerosis. But I had a nearly week-long trip beginning the next day with commitments in New York, Colorado Springs, and Houston. This year had been pretty tough on the family finances. My wife, Teresa, and I had labeled it the Financial Perfect Storm. Each one of these upcoming meetings was a step toward calming those waters. Push through the pain, I thought; you just don't have time to get sick. I told no one.

As I worked steadily through the day, the numbness dissipated and I convinced myself I was getting better. But once I was in New York, the headaches began: intense pressure behind my eyes that radiated pain through my shoulders. I was dosing myself with handfuls of over-the-counter headache remedies, pinching the web of my thumb in an attempt at self-acupressure, and struggling to sleep with a cold rag over my eyes. Nothing spelled relief.

Sleepless in New York, I caught a 6:00 A.M. flight to Colorado Springs. There I met my host, Dr. Jim Humphries, the veterinary contributor for CBS. Dr. Jim knew something was wrong and tried to get me to go to the emergency room. I persuaded him I was feeling much better and, after our meeting, he dropped me at the airport. At the airport I started to stumble. I called Dr. Steve Garner, a veterinary colleague and my friend of four years, whom I was flying to meet at his seminar in Houston. His alarm at my symptoms really shook me.

At the gate, my cell phone started going off. The first call was from Jim, who said he wasn't convinced I was improving. He wanted to come back and drive me to the emergency room, but I turned him down. Then Steve called to tell me he'd arranged for a friend of his, a neurologist at Baylor University, to see me as soon as I landed. How badly I wanted to go home. I slumped in a seat at the gate, cross-eyed with pain. I pictured Teresa and our children, daughter Mikkel, fourteen, and son Lex, ten, sitting, as we had so many evenings that summer, on the deck of our home in Bonners Ferry, Idaho, surrounded by pets. Our house looks down the throat of a thirty-mile-long glacial river valley. We like to watch the light fade in the evening as herds of deer, elk, and even the occasional moose migrate across the valley floor, while hawks and bald eagles swoop overhead. If I was this sick, I wanted that sight, those smells, my family. I called our family doctor, Dr. Will McCreight, who told me exactly what my heart was saying: come home.

I was on the jetway about to board the plane home when Steve called again. He'd talked to his neurologist friend who believed there might be bleeding in the lining around my brain. "Do not board the plane," he said. The change in pressure on the ascent might kill me. I should go immediately to a hospital in Colorado Springs. I told Steve I was going home, and stepped back from the stream of passengers to pray that I was making the right decision. Then I boarded. The anxiety I felt made the trip one of the longest of my life, but I made it. By the time I landed around eleven that night, Dr. McCreight had arranged for me to see a neurologist in Coeur d'Alene the next morning and booked an appointment for an MRI.

The doctor who examined me unsmilingly offered four possibilities: stroke, brain tumor, multiple sclerosis, or subarachnoid hemorrhage, the official name for bleeding between the linings around the brain. When I went in for the MRI, the staff cautioned me that the test was noisy and claustrophobic. Even some of the local miners got antsy in the MRI tunnel, they said. They asked if I'd like to listen to music during the full-body scan and I chose a CD of gospel hymns. Imagine my trepidation when the first soothing hymn had the lyrics, "Softly and tenderly Jesus is calling, come home, come home/Ye who are weary come home." Maybe I should have taken my second choice of Credence Clearwater Revival.

The MRI results were the best I could have hoped for, however. I had a simple mechanical problem—an intervertebral disc in my neck had prolapsed, spilling its contents onto my spinal cord. The discs that cushion the bones of your spine are constructed like a jelly donut: a harder core on the outside, with a softer, jellylike middle. Usually when a disc slips it affects only one side, but mine was more severe, putting extreme pressure across the whole cord. That was what had caused the bilateral numbness. The headaches were from muscle spasms and anxiety. I would need surgery to remove the damaged disc, during which they'd insert a poker chip-size piece of cow bone to keep the correct spacing and fuse the instability in my spine with a titanium plate. My doctor gave me some muscle relaxants for the anxiety and sent me home in a neck brace to await my appointment with the neurosurgeon, which couldn't be scheduled until the end of December, six long weeks away. In the meantime, he advised me to slow down and prepare for a lengthy recuperation.

Although I was relieved that the diagnosis wasn't any of the four conditions I'd feared, I still had a hard time accepting that I had to slow down. When we moved to Bonners Ferry five years earlier, Teresa had named our ranch Almost Heaven because she saw it as an oasis of beauty, goodness, and serenity. We designed family stationery and I added the slogan "Life in the slow lane." But the slogan had become a joke to my family. Ever since we arrived here, I'd worked even harder than before, all the while promising that I was just about to slow down. As soon as I finished one obligation or chased down another opportunity, another presented itself and I was off again. It always seemed more important to take care of business than to take care of myself. In fact, since we moved to this beautiful, peaceful place, I'd gained twenty-five pounds and had developed high blood pressure.

Teresa saw this crisis as an opportunity to force me to be true to my word. She begged me to look through my calendar for the next six months and start saying no to a number of things I'd said yes to. The mere suggestion of that caused me shame. What if I missed something? What if no one missed me? I started calling my friends and colleagues, bemoaning my fate, and in a way asking their permission to say no. Uniformly they told me to slow down and give myself a chance to heal.

Even as Teresa and I walked to the horse barn the next morning to do our chores for our quarter horses, Sugar Babe, Chex, Pegasus, and Gabriel, I was arguing with the prognosis. I'd always had perfect health and the capacity to dig deep and tough it out—the determination I'd called on as an athlete to play while hurt, or as a farm boy whose father needed the crops in before the storm hit, whether or not I had the flu. The doctor said I had to stay put for six weeks or more after the surgery, but I'd always been a fast healer. I'd probably be back up to speed in a month or less, I reasoned.

The horses were galloping in the paddock, anticipating their morning meal. Teresa rolled back the door to the barn to let them into their stalls as I got the pitchfork to hoist a briefcase-size piece of hay bale to feed them. I stuck the fork in and suddenly found that I just didn't have the strength to lift even that meager amount. Ashamed I couldn't complete a task I'd done regularly since I was about five or six, I struggled in silence, using all the tricks I'd learned as a farm kid ordered to hoist something heavier than me. Pride forced me to try, but pride alone couldn't get the bundle to move. I had to ask Teresa to do it for me.

The first snowfall that year was early and very wet, the kind of heavy, dense snow that makes great "soaker" snowballs but can be rough on horses' feet. I could see that our horses were walking gingerly from compacted balls of ice that had wedged right into the center of their hooves. At least I could help them with that, I thought. I got the long-handled screwdriver and leaned into the meat of Sugar Babe's right front leg, flexing her foot to rest it on my upper thigh. Another defeat. I choked up as I admitted to Teresa that I just didn't have the strength to do this, either. Again I had to ask my petite, five-foot, four-inch wife to perform a task I'd done a hundred times.

I held Sugar Babe's reins as Teresa worked on her hoof, but my mind was ten thousand feet above, lost in the profound identity crisis of illness. I saw myself as the endurance champ, the tireless provider. If I am not the things that I do—if I have to do different things and do things differently—who am I? The question was too frightening to answer. Sugar Babe laid her massive head on my shoulder with the gentleness of a baby's touch, and I reached up reflexively to stroke her muzzle. There are few things softer than a horse's muzzle, the animal equivalent of velvet. Horses take in the world through the mouth, and that supple, responsive muzzle serves as their fingers and hands. Sugar Babe pulled up a little and began nibbling over my neck with her vibrissae, tactile hairs similar to a cat's whiskers but of varied lengths and scattered across the surface of her nose and mouth. She roamed until she came to rest at the exact spot on my neck that hurt.

She still had a head of steam from her run in the paddock and her breath shot from her nostrils in forceful ostrich plumes. At 101.5 degrees Fahrenheit, a horse's body temperature is a few degrees higher than ours. Her hot breath on my neck in the cold barn was like a steam treatment. As she settled, I adjusted to the ebb and flow of her breath and felt myself relax for the first time since this soul-shaking experience. I was alive, with my loved ones, and I was home: three simple facts that I had taken for granted and that, as a result, were very nearly lost to me. In that simple way that animals have of bringing you back to your world, Sugar Babe was showing me that my healing would have to start here.

The feeling of Sugar Babe's laying on of hands through the gentle pressure of her muzzle on my neck stuck with me as Teresa and I walked back to the house. Truly I had a burden that was too heavy for me to carry, something that couldn't be shoved aside by cleverness and dogged determination. As uncomfortable as the idea made me, I had to look at this illness not as a defeat, but as a gift—a chance to repot, renew, recharge myself. The first thing that had to go was the stress.

Teresa and I took out my schedule for the next six months and made a list of all the engagements I'd have to cancel. Once the schedule was clear, we blocked off a lot of family time. Teresa didn't stop at just the visible stress. I have a drawer in my office that is filled to the top with things I want to find a way to do, such as chairing fund-raisers, making speeches, leading the charge for causes, or reviewing a colleague's manuscript. That drawer was now too heavy for me to lift. Teresa took the drawer and ceremoniously dumped its contents straight into the trash. Then she asked for a very specific Christmas present. She begged me to lose twenty-five pounds and get control of my blood pressure.

Lessening stress creates a different kind of anxiety. What exactly was I supposed to do with myself? The cliché "Physician heal thyself" took on an ironic twist for me. I've been a pet lover and animal lover my whole life, and have observed countless times in my years as a practicing veterinarian how a strong relationship with animals often gives people the strength and motivation to reclaim their health after an illness knocks them down. I've spent my professional life celebrating this special relationship that we call "the Bond," the healthy, affection connection between people and their pets that science is only now beginning to appreciate fully. Yet I'd never been really sick; never had to call on pets to point me toward a healthier lifestyle. This Bond that I could describe in passionate detail I'd only felt as an observer. In reality, I didn't have the first idea about how to heal.

My own words rattled around in my head: the stories, studies, and statistics that I'd often cited to demonstrate the healing power of pets for a host of dire medical conditions. For instance, those who have animals in their homes have an eight times greater chance of surviving one year after a heart attack. Pets lessen stress by lowering heart rate, blood pressure, and even cholesterol. Those with pets have fewer doctor visits, shorter hospital stays, and an easier time adapting to a new routine of recuperation after an illness. Pets combat depression and isolation through their role as a social ice breaker, giving others something to talk about besides the illness. Most important, the physicality of the relationship with an animal is a boon to health. The healing touch of petting an animal and being kissed or nuzzled in return establishes a soothing intimacy at a time of loneliness. They also serve as a stimulus to exercise, a key factor in most recuperation. But the element of this powerful relationship that had always impressed me the most was the importance of nurturing another creature. At a time when the ill person is feeling disconnected from the world, incapable of his or her normal responsibilities, the pet demonstrates that they are still needed by another and that their presence would be terribly missed.

If you had asked me about the Bond I had with our animals, I'd have rated our relationship a ten. All of our pets have carefully monitored diets, regular checkups by the in-house vet, ample opportunity for exercise, and they are surrounded by a family who loves and pampers them. Yet my illness revealed to me that, like so many things I cherished in life, I had the time now, if I could find the patience, to simply watch the animals with an eye to understanding the way they could nurture me. As I began to focus on the world in front of my face, not three thousand miles beyond, I began to find this nurturing in every interaction, even in something as simple as coming home.

My family usually knows within minutes what time I'll be dropping off that mountain road for the final eighth-of-a-mile plunge down the driveway to our log house. If it is the middle of the night and Teresa, Mikkel, and Lex are enveloped deep within their goose-down comforters, I don't expect them to leave their warm beds to greet me. But I could also be coming home at 6:00 P.M. with nothing good on television and no phone ringing, and they still don't rush out to greet me. Not once have I made the final turn to see Teresa bound across the yard in slow motion, romance novel fashion, for a leap-into-your-arms greeting. Never have I slowed to pull into the garage and noted Mikkel and Lex's faces pressed to the glass of the windows aglow with delight and hands waving.

But 24/7, in all weather conditions, without a day off for sleeping in or because they just don't feel like it, Sirloin, our black Labrador retriever, and LLLucky, our wonder dog (as in "I wonder what kind of dog he is?"), are waiting, agog with anticipation. They twitch on the grass launching pad in the middle of our circular driveway like two teapots that are ready to blow, waiting for the moment when I finally stop the vehicle and step out of the car.

Three-legged LLLucky always wins the race to greet me, advancing recklessly with his bark sounding out like a bass drum. Four-legged and fleet, Sirloin is delayed because his retriever background won't allow him to approach me without bringing an offering in the form of a disarticulated skeleton from the woods, a stick, a toy, a pine cone, whatever. With curled tails sweeping rhythmically from side to side, mouths open with silly grins, they collide into my body in a delighted frenzy of fur. Scooter, sleeping under six inches of goose down in Mikkel's room, is nowhere to be seen.

Then it's my turn. With a high-pitched voice that is only activated by our daily reunions, I call their names and nicknames, as I search out their favorite places to be scratched or rubbed. "Gomer, youzzzz Daddy's *big* boy, aren't you," I whine and coo as I scratch the inside of Sirloin's pendulous ears. "Boo let the dogs out, hoo, hoo, hoo, hoo," I chant to LLLucky, who we sometimes call Boo, in our family's parody of the 2000 hit song from Baja Men. These are unique nicknames and this is a special voice I have for no other creatures in the world.

When I look into their dancing liquid eyes filled with love, I don't know whether they shine for me or the can opener. But I really don't care. I only know that I feel the stresses of the outside world slipping away, the ritual instantly connecting me back to simple pleasures, with no expectations of my performance.

Some summer nights when I come home, rather than simply placating the dogs and heading into the house, we lie out on the grass and gaze into the sky. Sirloin and LLLucky brace me, following the movements of my head as I do a slow scan above. The stars pierce the Crayola black sky, and shooting stars sometimes sweep from the top of one mountain range to the other, leaving a trail of luminescent dust to mark the path. Because of this downtime, literally, I know the phases of the moon, many of the constellations, the routes of satellites, where the North Star is tethered that night, the sounds of the nocturnal world providing the most soothing background music imaginable.

That was what they could bring more of to me: the moment of joy, the point of connection, a call to take a long look at the beauty of the life around me. Through all of these gifts, the animals could help me heal. Every step I took toward improving their lives, I slowly began to realize, was a step toward better health and happiness for me. I'm a man who is used to broad strokes, big gestures, quick hits, in and out. Knowing that you've left a mark, but not staying long enough to see the ripple effect. At a time when I wasn't feeling so effective in the world, they could guide me to being effective in a smaller, simpler way in the immediate circle around me. They could demonstrate how to have this power in the intimate realm, to touch it in a way that is sustaining and beneficial not just to the animals but to my whole family.

When you look at them gathered in a ragged trio, our three dogs don't exactly look like physician's assistants, physical therapists, or shrinks, but that's just what they became for me. I was soon to experience the fact that animal rescues don't necessarily have to come in the form of a dog dragging you from a burning building to qualify as heroic. Just as often, pets perform heroic rescues on a daily basis, just by being there during times of need.

Scooter is our beloved and somewhat bloated wirehaired fox terrier. A classic terrier, she's full of energy, irrepressible, and pugnacious, her expression alert and fiery. We lovingly call her "the hairy princess" to mark her royal status as the family's sole indoor dog and her uncanny ability to work around our "no-treat" policy. She's got a wide variety of canine accouterments, such as a hand-woven collar, seasonal bandannas, even an Elvis outfit complete with dog-size guitar.

Seeing her as a princess, I never expected her to be focused on the needs of others. Yet during my recovery from spinal surgery, Scooter drew even closer to me. In those tough weeks between my diagnosis and the date of my surgery, I spent a lot of time on the couch, remote in hand, with my body propped up like I was in the space shuttle ready for launch—pillows under my neck and a stack three deep under my knees. She would come up to the couch and lift my numb right hand with her Jimmy Durante snout, letting me know that she was lying there at my side if I needed her.

As much as I drew on Scooter's model of forbearance with grace, I marveled at LLLucky's cheerful personality despite his own disability. Nobody can resist LLLucky, whose multiple L's mark his three narrow escapes with death before he became a member of our family. Born into a house devoid of love or even simple kindness, his owner had chosen him in hopes that the German shepherd part of his pedigree would render him a macho, aggressive guard dog. No matter what abuse he suffered— even losing his front right leg in a battle with a freight train—the stalwart animal maintained his gentle demeanor. When I first saw LLLucky, his stump of a left front leg was still swollen from the surgery performed to remove the crushed fragments of bone and detritus. His face was bike wreck raw from having slid down the highway at 65 mph. Even his intact right front paw had a toe that was cherry tomato red, grotesquely swollen, and infected.

LLLucky typified what I'd seen so many times before as a veterinarian. Not weighted down by self-consciousness, seeking no sympathy, and unwilling to "dog it," pets bounce back from major accidents or illnesses like superballs. For LLLucky, losing his leg or flying out of the rescue vehicle for a three-point crash landing was more like removing a splinter than a leg. According to our veterinarian, Dr. Rolan Hall, who treated LLLucky after the accidents, never once did he whine, cry out in pain, or quit wagging his tail. He simply wanted food (and lots of it because he'd been starved) and a little love. Now that he has both in abundance at our home, he's always joyous and uncomplaining. His puppy playfulness belies his Abe Lincoln-like adult face. Despite missing a front leg, he manages bursts of speed and agility that astonish our guests.

Through the example of their love and personal courage, Scooter and LLLucky helped show me the more private and spiritual aspects of healing the mind and the spirit. Equally important was gradually using my body more and more. This is where our black Lab, Sirloin, volunteered for duty.

We joke that four-year-old Sirloin is two neurons connected to a set of teeth. He moves through the world without the burden of hate, bitterness, or jealousy, his tail wagging in perpetual motion.

I've had Labs since I was a young boy on the farm. To me, they are proof positive that Mother Nature does indeed play favorites. These versatile animals are in demand as guide dogs for the blind, drug-sniffing dogs, gun dogs, and as reliable family pets. They are gentle, loyal, even-tempered, intelligent, and eager to please.

Sirloin has the genes of a champion. His father was a renowned canine athlete in field trials, and he is so beautifully contoured and chiseled with muscle that a visitor to Almost Heaven Ranch commented that he looked like he could be Michelangelo's *David*'s dog.

So here I had three creatures living in the full range of health: Sirloin in his prime, plucky LLLucky disabled but undaunted, and geriatric Scooter ailing but never failing. At the same time that I was trying to re-create myself, I decided to try to figure out what the next phase of their lives would be like. I wanted to give Scooter relief, as I now knew how much her arthritis must hurt. I wanted LLLucky to know that he would never be hungry, cold, or alone again—that he was in the safety of the loving arms of our family for as long as he lived. The best gift I could give Sirloin was full vitality, the chance to use the abilities languishing in his genes. Relief, comfort, and vitality are a pretty good description of what I also wanted for myself. I began to see that every way I had of strengthening the Bond was actually a step toward my own recovery.

In the course of paying more attention to the dogs, a much deeper level of communication, trust, and interaction developed between us. I watched the way our dogs and cats carried their ears, moved their tails, and the way their expressive eyes were picture windows into their hearts and heads. Veterinary ethologist Myrna Milani told me that dogs could understand 180 human words, something I found remarkable. Even more remarkable was her follow-up question: How many different barks or meows do you recognize?

Over time and with study and careful attention, I found I could recognize a lot. I looked deeply into their dark eyes to see if they were shining with the anticipation of play or a treat, or with delight about the FedEx truck coming down the road. I could tell if their eyes were dulled with the pain of arthritis, or filled with sadness over an empty food bowl. Sometimes I could see that they were clouded with confusion over "who's in charge here?": it was a much different look than one of dreamy-eyed satisfaction. With the flick of a tail, a silly grin, a bark or meow, rubbing against me, or locking on eye-to-eye, encyclopedic amounts of information were being communicated that I had previously missed.

The first day of January 2001, just four days after having my neck fused, on my doctor's orders and to fulfill my promised Christmas present for Teresa, I started morning sessions on the treadmill. Teresa is the type who can pound away happily for hours on those machines, but for me, half an hour of forced labor is about my limit. So each afternoon I began taking walks accompanied by Sirloin, my own personal rehab Lab.

My first tentative outing was only the distance from our house to the barn, about the length of a soccer field. I'd forgotten that this is how everyone has to start toward a goal.

One step at a time.

Up to the barn and back.

Then up to the barn and back twice. A week later, past the barn, down the hill, and back. Movement was painful, and the route we took was repetitive at first. I viewed it as a duty, and when I said to Sirloin: "C'mon, let's go for our walk," the tone was less joyful and more dirge-like. But as my strength and stability improved, I decided to stop being in charge and just to follow Sirloin.

My walk was transformed by piggybacking on his acute senses. When I looked at the trail I saw nothing, but through him I saw every-thing. It was amazing to watch him alert to movement hundreds of yards away, something I normally would have been blind to. Or to have him screech to a halt, nose down, detecting the presence of a bird that had walked by many minutes ago.

Soon shuffling steps turned into long strides over varied terrain as the days turned into weeks. With Sirloin in the lead, we traveled up mountains, down wooded ravines, and through streambeds in pursuit of quarry to which we meant no harm. There were times when I'd be crawling on my hands and knees through the brush to explore Sirloin's latest prized discovery, such as a pile of fresh deer dung. We fed our spirits by resting on the rocks and reveling in the splendor of northern Idaho.

In just three months, I knocked twenty-five pounds off my frame and actually had pants that didn't fit like a tourniquet. My back stopped hurting from carrying a large fanny pack in the form of an actual fanny. My fused neck could once again swivel as I viewed the panorama of sky and mountain. The fresh air, peace, and beauty of my environment, as well as the loving canine companionship and vigorous exercise, were transforming me. For the first time in more years than I can remember, I was off the road to ruin and on the road to health.

But Sirloin's gift to me was so much more generous than that. Through his intense focus on his surroundings, he lent me the capacity we modern humans so envy: the ability to be completely in the present. When I'm focusing on Sirloin, I'm not thinking about what I'm going to do when I get back; he's not thinking about next year or how to realize his full Lab potential. He's not even thinking, really. He's much too fascinated by the world right under his nose.

Sirloin wanted to fetch. He'd bring me little totems of affection such as pinecones or sticks and waggle them around his mouth, taunting me to grab them away from him. In the beginning I'd turn him down. I was too focused on getting in my daily ration of exercise to appreciate the gift he was offering me. My notion of play was stuck in the narrow version of the human world. When you play with a fellow human, you play to win. Either you want to win, or at the very least, you don't want to look stupid. But with a pet, the point of play is to engage. Your cat will swipe at that piece of yarn for as long as you want. She'll even let you have it sometimes. And your dog will happily fetch that stick until you're both exhausted. No hidden agendas, no posturing for personal gain, no duplicity. Just play for the sake of play.

When doctors recommend that patients get an animal for exercise, they rarely recommend a cat, because the accepted wisdom is that cats just can't be bothered. One of the most used books on my shelf is *The Perfect Puppy*. But let me tell you, the book has no counterpart in the feline world. Despite our attempts to make everything march at a pace commensurate with the urgency of our lives, cats have flat-out refused to toe the line, or even approach it, for that matter. Unlike dogs, who have been likened to people in fur coats, cats are proud members of another species who at best tolerate our whims.

While other domesticated species are sociable by nature, the cat typically walks a fine line between being aloof and alone, and sociable on its own timing and terms, thinking primarily of its own comforts. For many cat lovers like myself, it is the unpredictability, solitary nature, and preoccupation with self that makes it such an attractive pet partner. One of my favorite cat books is *Cats for Dummies*—and that about sums up most of our knowledge about these incredible creatures. That's why, when embarking on my self-improvement campaign, I didn't at first consider our barn cats, Turbo and Tango, as allies.

We always had a variety of toys for the cats to play with—catnip toys, plastic balls trapped in circular tracks, bells—but I'd never taken a dedicated approach to getting them to play. And as a vet, I usually brushed aside clients' requests for games to take weight off of a fat cat, because I thought nothing much worked. But as I opened myself to the world that was obvious to my dogs, I became just as curious about life with the cats and what delights they might offer.

Turbo and Tango have lived their whole lives in and around our horse barn. North Idaho seasons can be harsh, so trips to the barn are often a sprint before the birds are even up to take care of the animals' basic needs: get them food and make sure the water isn't frozen. We'd stand in the doorway of the feed room/cat bedroom and call Turbo and Tango down from the loft, then hurriedly shut the door behind them, taking comfort in knowing that they were safe from predators and out of the elements. While the animals ate, we'd open up the barn and look down the valley to see if a storm was lurking over the nearby mountains. The basic needs of all the animals have always been taken care of, but I would check them off like tasks in a day planner. I felt Turbo and Tango had pretty good lives, all things considered. They had a huge warm barn as their personal playground, one that was amply stocked with prey for them to chase and conquer. As with the other animals, I didn't think I could make their lives much better until I stopped to really look.

Yet when I did, I found out that play for them is not simply a medley of infantile behavior, but an extremely complex phenomenon, because it is free and variable, and not constrained by rigid patterns. Play introduces novelty into behavior, continuously providing the cats opportunities to learn, and to use latent skills.

I went to Petco and bought a sample of almost every cat toy they had. I had feathers attached to fishing poles, wind-up mice, even high-tech toys like laser pointers. At times Teresa and I got more exercise out of the toys than Turbo and Tango, who frequently showed disinterest and disdain for our new purchases. But other times, after shuffling through toys like Las Vegas blackjack dealers, we'd find the perfect toy for that moment and would be laughing, hitting each other on the arm, and saying, "Did you see that?" winding up a mechanical mouse while simultaneously winding down.

I took the lessons I learned from my healing and looked at my relationships with my children. We are a close family, a family of strong traditions, rituals, and bonds held in place by a shared faith. I was willing to bet there were subtleties I was missing in my relationship with my children and that it could be dramatically improved, as well. In a contradiction of the old saying, I wanted to treat my kids like the dogs, and they'd be better for it.

My son, Lex, is obsessed with a military strategy game called War Hammer. A cross between checkers and chess, it is an intricate game with warships, weapons, and soldiers, and a rule book the size of the Manhattan phone book. I've always felt that if there are rules, I want to follow them. Keep score, play to win, follow the fine print to the letter. Lex wanted to make the rules up, to freelance, to use his imagination. He even wanted to change them in the middle of his turn. What would start off as a time for us to be together would frequently end in a squabble because I thought he was trying to gain an unfair advantage over me by changing the rules. My parental voice would intone that rules needed to be obeyed if he was going to learn how to succeed in the bigger game of life. One day after a beautiful walk with Sirloin, I decided to let Lex change the rules ad nauseam; focus on his love of the game and time together, and not on the outcome or final score.

It was euphoria for Lex. He got so excited because I focused my complete attention and spirit on him. He'd make a move in the game and I'd say, "Gosh darn, I knew you were going to get me." He taunted me during the game and squealed at a great move, whether it was his or mine. High-fives turned into mock disgust when I did my special dice-throwing chant or danced as I destroyed one of his armies. I found I had a special voice for Lex, different from the one I had for the dogs. Lex came upstairs, his face beaming, his voice hoarse from screaming, but still able to chatter endlessly about the game, transformed by our spontaneity into a lasting memory.

With an adolescent girl such as my daughter, it's a little harder to find a way to connect. They have so much more of their lives that they want to keep private that you walk a fine line between encouragement and intrusion. Mikkel has talents she wants to use, much like Sirloin has, and I'm trying in my way to help her develop. I go with her to her singing lessons and film her. I make it more of a priority to really attend to the performance, playing it back and giving her feedback in a way that supports her growth and builds her strength. That nurtures her and the life of our family, as much as it nurtures me.

Our society seems fixated on the miracle machine or wonder drug that can effortlessly prolong lives. Being disease-free is only one measurement of health, as my illness so dramatically demonstrated to me. The World Health Organization defines health as: "A state of complete physical, mental, and social well-being, and not merely the absence of disease or infirmity." To have a life worth living, you need to connect to those around you and contribute to their lives. This is where the Bond plays such a crucial role. At a time when psychology, sociology, and politics have sucked the spontaneity out of human relations, the simplicity of our affection with pets is a model for the smaller, intimate moments that really sustain us. Without those ties that bind—the bonds of love, friendship, responsibility, and dependence—we gradually begin to wither away. It is our bonds that keep us healthy.

I believe that pets prolong our lives by reacquainting us with our animal nature, the elemental self that our society and lifestyle conspire to suppress. When we talk about someone's animal nature, the qualities that first come to mind are brutal, sexual, and vicious; yet these qualities are only intermittently present in the animal world. Through a close relationship with our pets, we awaken the other equally powerful animal traits of loyalty, love, physicality, and playfulness.

Against the backdrop of forced and awkward contact with the world, the regularity of that wagging tail and the unconditional affection of your pets brings you instantly out of isolation. You stop rattling around inside your own head, and focus on what they give you—simply and for free. If I walk out of the house and ask Sirloin if he wants to go up to the horse barn, there is no way he's going to say, "No, not today. You go without me." He's perpetually convinced that this is the greatest idea anyone has ever had.

Now I know the exact spot on the gravel path where he turns back to look at me and reinforce his enthusiasm for the one hundred-yard walk. I also can trace the precise route he takes as he sniffs around the barn to make sure everything is in order while I do my horse-tending chores. We've done this together a thousand times, but since I got ill, this never fails to remind me to slow down and cherish the rituals of everyday life.

Of course, every day is full of ritualized activity. You get up at a certain time, start the coffee before breakfast, and take your shower after a prescribed series of actions, all of which you perform as a mindless routine. A conscious ritual recognizes the values and intentions that underpin our lives. Prior to my illness, I sometimes saw my tasks at the horse barn as boring, taking too much of my valuable time. Now when Sirloin takes that turn on the pathway and lavishes on me a bit of his joy, or when the cats leap from fence post to fence post to shadow me as I clean out the corral, I feel my connection to our pets, our animal neighbors, nature, and my family's pleasure and pride in the horses. I inhale a breath of my good fortune in having these people and pets in my life, and breathe in the beauty of life itself. And while Sirloin is just being his happy dog self, he reminds me of the reason I do the things I do, and the meaning beneath even the smallest action.

In the last twenty years, medical research has detailed the soothing effect pets have on the elderly, the stressed, and the emotionally disengaged. The other health benefits of pets only become apparent when you get sick. A study of postoperative heart patients conducted by doctors from Duke University found that those accustomed to the routine of caring for a pet had an easier time adjusting to the new rigors of self-care, which in many cases facilitated a speedier and more complete recovery. Elderly people who have pet companions have a lower incidence of cancer, studies find, but pets can be helpful to people of any age who have contracted the disease. Mayo Clinic oncologist Dr. Edward T. Creagan has found pets to be so beneficial to health that he prescribes them as part of treatment for a third of his patients. In fact, scientists find that pets can prevent, detect, help treat, and in some cases cure a variety of maladies.

Animal trainer Duane Pickel taught his championship bomb-sniffing schnauzer George to detect human time bombs—melanomas that are too small to be found by the human eye. He was prompted to try by the urging of Dr. Armand Cognetta, a Tallahassee, Florida, dermatologist who was growing increasingly discouraged by the tools available for detecting skin cancer. The incidence of skin cancer is on the rise nationally, and early detection is the best way to affect a cure. Even though Dr. Cognetta examined his patients with a handheld microscope, he was only able to find 80 percent of the melanomas in time.

Then he found Duane Pickel, who has trained the bomb-sniffing dogs for the Reagan and Bush Senior administrations. George was his most honored dog, holding the world record for sniffing out bombs in competition. Dr. Cognetta got melanoma tissue samples from a local research hospital, and Duane worked with George to hone his nose for cancer. When Dr. Cognetta found patients willing to be sniffed by George, he discovered skin cancers on four out of seven of them.

Medicine today often chases after a disease with a treatment when it's too late to reverse the damage to the body. Doctors, limited by their human senses in what they can detect, wait for a symptom to present and then react. With most illnesses, that detection is limited to what can be seen with the eyes. Pickel believes that dogs potentially could be trained to detect the onset of many diseases with their superior sense of smell. The scientific community has been so intrigued by George's results that researchers at the Smithsonian Institute have embarked on projects related to George's groundbreaking results.

Besides cancer detection, pets can help treat a whole host of chronic conditions that lead to severe health problems. Some of the most stressed-out people in the world are stockbrokers, living at a frantic pace as they respond quickly to the most subtle shift or precipitous drop in the market. They are perfect candidates for heart attacks, and many of them are on medication for hypertension. A study of New York City stockbrokers who were taking medication for hypertension conducted by Dr. Karen Allen of the State University of New York at Buffalo, found that once the stockbrokers brought a pet into their homes, their stress levels dropped dramatically. Nearly half of them were able to go off their medication. In fact, just having a pet in the room—even a tank full of fish—makes people feel safer and calmer, as studies in doctors' waiting rooms have demonstrated.

Simple weekly visits from pets have had remarkable success in bringing Alzheimer's sufferers and autistic children back to reality, stimulating them to smile, touch, laugh, and talk. Caring for an animal, whether it is prisoners training service dogs for the disabled or children with Attention Deficit Disorder tending hamsters, acquaints people with respect, self-control, and responsibility. In none of these cases are people "cured" by their pets, but pets reach them in ways that traditional medications and humans cannot. As a result of their relationship with animals, these people become more attentive and responsive citizens of the world, more aware of the needs of others, and more responsible for their own behavior, which is just this side of a miracle.

For all these reasons—social, emotional, physical—this is a Bond worth exploring, celebrating, protecting, and expanding. I believe that if people had the right pets for their needs, this world would be a happier, healthier place. If you are inspired by the stories you read in this book to consider adding a four-legged member to the family, that's great, but it's not a decision to be made lightly.

So many animals end up in shelters because there's a fad for Taco Bell Chihuahuas or Disney dalmatians, but the breed characteristics or needs—nervousness or a desire to run—don't match those of the owner. Or they are drawn to cuddling a kitten, but don't know how to raise a cat. I'm going to offer guidance on picking the right breed for your expectations, lifestyle, and resources.

Strengthening the Bond is our responsibility as the caretakers of the animal world. Medicine is medicine, whether for a cat or a cow or a human. The tests to diagnose illnesses are the same and doctors researched most medicines on animals first, so they work across the species. As animals' role as companions has taken precedence over utility, we treat pets less like property and recognize their personalities. As a result, we're willing to spend more to keep them around. Twenty years ago if a dog got cancer, you put him down. Now cancer treatment and hip replacement surgery for pets is commonplace, leading to a trend toward merging the two medical disciplines. Universities in Colorado, Michigan, and Missouri are integrating their veterinary and human medical programs, and many others are considering the possibilities.

These new medical alliances are practical in more than just a bureaucratic sense. Taking better care of our companions can encourage us to be more healthy. People are very regular in keeping up the yearly physical and the vaccinations for their animals, but can go decades without checking on their own health. All medically trained people—including vets—should encourage their patients to get examined regularly. And in treating chronic conditions, the cross-species connection can be emphasized for mutual health. If the owner is a couch potato, so is his pet, and the lifestyle changes necessary to prolong the life of the human are the same for the animal, too.

What I hope you'll find in this book is not just a connection, but an opportunity. If we use our reason, logic, and dexterity to stamp out illnesses, we create a healthy environment for all creatures. In return, our pets give us their absolute all. This is without a doubt the best deal mankind has ever made. This vital link to the world fuels our spirit, supplies passion to our lives, and makes us laugh. It is the Bond to God, to animals, to nature, and to other people. It is the common fiber of a happy, healthy person and one of society's major weapons against loneliness, lethargy, and depression. Our beloved pets are like vitamins fortifying us against invisible threats: like seat belts cradling against life's crashes; like alarm systems giving us a sense of security. Taken together, the healing power of pets is powerful medicine indeed.

PART ONE

The Healing
Power of Pets

A Healthy Start—
The Power of Childhood Pets

WHEN I LECTURE ABOUT THE Bond, I try to cut away the lofty phrases and go right to the heart by asking people to describe their childhood pets. Even in dignified places of learning such as the Smithsonian Institution, the knitted brows smooth and smiles spread across the faces of nearly everyone in the room. Their shoulders drop as their minds travel back to a time ten to sixty years past. They're getting off the bus from school and their dogs are running full-tilt to greet them. They're under a shade tree nestled in the deep grass just before mowing, sneaking their dog a morsel from yesterday's dinner. Or they're patting the cover with two hands, trying to determine which of the lumps is the cat.

People remember the relationship with their first pet as taking place in a simpler time in their lives, even though most of what you go through growing up is far from simple. As kids, we try to find a pattern in all of the stimuli, decide what to trust and what to fear, and along the way experience our first joy, connection, rejection, loneliness, and heartbreak. We face some of our largest challenges and most memorable triumphs. Frequently, the companionship of pets is the constant that gets us through.

I grew up on a small family farm in southern Idaho—160 acres— and you almost had to break the back of the farm to support a family of six from that amount of land. The machine was at full throttle all the time, from the first row of sugar beets planted in March to the last row of potatoes harvested in October. We were the picture of the hard-working family farm that people romanticize today as agribusiness gobbles up the landscape. That romantic picture misses the incredible stress of battling the uncertainties that those who work the land face: weather, weeds, water, insects, yields, and commodity prices.

Daily my dad wore that stress on his face as he scanned the fields with a critical eye. Our farm was on a flat table of desert land, and if in early March my father spotted a cloud of dust moving on the horizon, he'd nearly twitch in his skin from anxiety. Some other farmer was working his fields before my father. Some other farmer might be getting an edge, or maybe had heard something Dad hadn't about the weather or the water. In the days before herbicides, his crew of field hands—my mother, three siblings, and I—could be called away from whatever we were doing if he happened to spy rogue plants in the field. Even our Sunday drives after church offered a chance to assess the state of the competition. "Bob, either you're going to drive the car or look at the fields, but you're not going to do both. You'll kill us all!" my mother would shriek as we wove down both lanes of the two-lane highway, ten miles an hour under the speed limit, with my father commenting on who wasn't watering enough or who needed to use more fertilizer.

As a lippy twelve-year-old, I boasted that I could be a better farmer than my father if I only had the chance. My father, to my surprise, took me up on the bet. He found me a piece of fallow pastureland to lease for only a thousand dollars a year, and cosigned for a two-thousand-dollar loan so I could also buy bean and grain seeds and fertilizer. Then he left me to make good on the challenge.

One February afternoon, I surveyed my little piece of earth with sinking spirits as Luke, my Labrador retriever shadow, sniffed the ground eagerly. I crouched on one knee and crumbled a handful of freeze-dried soil. How could I even match my father's yields on earth like this? And the fences—one of them five feet high, ten yards wide, and three hundred yards long—were made entirely of rocks pulled from this land, land that hadn't been farmed in twenty years or watered in three. By the time I got all the rocks out, I'd be able to build a fence of my own.

I cursed my father's name all spring as I worked that land, rooting out thousands of baseball- to basketball-size rocks and prying out one-hundred-pound ones with a crowbar. On the tractor, I could hear my father's insistence on ruler-straight rows, the farmer's equivalent of six-pack abs, as the spring-loaded plow ricocheted like a bumper car over rocks snagged in the plowshares. I'd get so frustrated, I'd kick the soil as I walked the boundaries of the fields. And so angry that I could cry at the impossibility of this dare. I don't know how I'd have done it without Luke.

For Luke, it was all an adventure. All I'd have to say is "load up," and he'd vault over the tailgate of the pickup truck, ready for the seven-mile ride from our farm to mine. When I was on the tractor tilling the soil or making small ditches to route the gravity-fed water, Luke would follow me up and back, resting only when I would. We'd walk the canal banks together, me in hip boots in the waist-deep water, sparks flying from my shovel blade as I chiseled slots into the rocky ground to divert water with canvas dams. Merrily he mirrored my every movement as he bounded, "Lab-happy," along the banks at my eye level. After all, there were flocks of pheasants to track over the land, burrowing owls that needed to be flushed from their holes, and a trout-filled spring whose water exited the earth at a refreshing 57 degrees.

So I planted my beans in rows twenty-two inches apart and drilled my barley seed, praying all the time that the soil had some power. As it turned out, the land was dense with micronutrients from the decades it had spent as pasture for cattle. My beans sprang up luxuriant, loaded with pods, and the gap between the rows closed a full ten days before my father's did. And the grain came up with heads thicker than the hair on a dog's back and as long as its tail.

My father took a long look around every time he dropped Luke and me off in the pickup, but he never said a word about how it was coming along. I knew he wouldn't speak too soon. Things sometimes took a sudden turn for the worse. Just the year before, he'd put in a field of high-priced garden beans so beautiful that neighbors stopped by to compliment him, jokingly calling him Jack (as in Jack and the Beanstalk) because the stalks were so thick and tall. We called them cougar beans for the royal blue Mercury Cougar we'd already picked out and were going to buy with the profit from this bin-busting bumper crop. But a week before harvest, the State of Idaho agricultural inspector discovered that they carried a virulent and contagious strain of halo blight. He ordered my father to plow the whole field under. The next day, our new Cougar was buried under the rolling earth of the plow. When it came to yields, there really wasn't much worth saying until the harvest. "Underpromise and overdeliver," my dad would say.

By September, the score was in. We went into Rangen's, the local feed and seed store, to have our crops weighed, cleaned, and stored for future sale. When I got out of the truck on the scales to pick up my weight tickets, the whole place was buzzing about my incredible yields. From the amount of land I worked, the average farmer would expect to get 20 one-hundred-pound sacks of beans and 80 bushels of grain per acre. My dad's yields always were among the very best, and this year he had 30 sacks of beans and 120 bushels of barley. But I'd doubled the average and even beaten my father by 30 percent, with 40 sacks of beans and 165 bushels of barley per acre. Still, he said nothing. He stood beside me while I soaked up the praise and capped it with his one and only compliment: "That Marty. He's something else. A real go-getter."

For a time I was mad at my dad for his underreaction to my achievement, but as I get older I understand that there are a lot of different facings to a memory. Sure, when I look back I see the sweat and the anger. I also see the pride and the triumph. The thread through it all is Luke. I see us splashing in the spring after a dusty afternoon of adding rocks to the great wall, or him jousting with our herd of Holstein steers, who followed us around like golden retrievers on hooves. I also remember like a photograph Luke's face when I presented him with the cow leg bone I'd bought him at the butcher shop at Rangen's to celebrate our yields, a bone so heavy he had to drag it around the ranch by one end. My father had an idea of how hard I'd worked, but Luke experienced it all. Luke, like so many people's childhood pets, lent a golden tone to the memory of some of life's harshest episodes: we shared the good and bad with a beloved animal companion who never disappointed and always validated.

Although estimates vary, surveys say that somewhere around 80 percent of families acquire some kind of pet during their children's tender years, often when children are between the ages of five and twelve. Studies show that the parents believe pets will foster sensitivity, responsibility, and will provide companionship—and their instincts are correct.

Children who help raise animals are better at decoding body language and understanding others' feelings and motives; what psychologists call empathy. Pet-owning children also score higher on nurturing. Even boys, who begin to abandon their softer side as they get into middle childhood, find no gender conflict in caring for animals. Before they are capable of giving to another person, very young children can get tremendous benefits from their relationships with animals. Recent studies show that they can help not only in early cognitive development, but also later help boost IQ scores, and can be part of improving a child's reading scores.

Child psychologist Foster Cline, who lives quite near me in Idaho, asks the joking question: "What of God's creatures is dumber than a newborn?" After all, they're not housebroken, he points out, and they don't have much motor control. He conjectures that a thoughtful boll weevil or a wise ant could easily outperform the average infant.

But babies are on an incredible learning curve. They enter the world with minds hungry to understand similarity and difference. Swiss developmentalist Jean Piaget, who studied the way children learn, divided their mental maturation into four stages, each building on the last. In the first stage of sensory motor development, their eyes are attracted by a shading of light, unexpected movements and their nervous systems crave new tactile sensations. Before they can form thoughts, they make sense literally through their senses. Each interaction with the material around them adds to their knowledge of how the world works and their place in it. They learn about their relationship to objects, how they move, and how to manipulate them and themselves. The very aliveness of animals stimulates babies to joyous interaction. It's what Harvard zoology Prof. Edward O. Wilson defined as biophilia: our innate tendency to focus on life and the lifelike processes, which he believes is central to our mental development.

On a research trip for this book, I was walking down a corridor in the University of Utah Hospital in Salt Lake City with Kathy McNulty and her ninety-pound akita Kyoshi, a much-honored animal assistance therapy dog. As we passed a waiting room, I glimpsed a young mother tending her toddler, a little girl who to all appearances had just started to walk. She was moving hand over hand around the lounge furniture, earnestly babbling away to her mom until the moment her eyes locked on Kyoshi. Then she got the look that kids of all ages get when they see an animal: the jaw drops down and they emit a sharp noise as they move toward their object of desire. In this case, the little girl walked like Frankenstein leaving the lab. Her legs thrust out stiffly and her footing was wobbly. Her arms stretched straight out in front. But unlike the Frankenstein coma stroll, this little girl's hands were palms up and open, and she was grinning as hard as she could grin, hoping for the chance to touch the incredible creature that had just passed.

Kyoshi, Kathy, and I were trotting down the hall to an appointment when the little girl's shriek stopped us in our tracks. The girl had made it all the way into the hallway unassisted (followed at a respectful distance by her mom) and was indignant that the prize she had worked so hard to obtain was slipping away. We walked back to the little girl, who buried her face in Kyoshi's long, buoyant fur with an exclamation of delight. The two creatures found themselves nose to nose. She patted Kyoshi's snout gently as it wriggled and snorted, exploring the scents of her face and shoulders. After elaborate good-byes, we left her standing in the hallway talking to her mother, presumably about the dog.

Many things in a child's world offer opportunities to understand similarity and difference, but, as Purdue University professor of child development Gail Melson puts it, animals are densely packed with information. Infants are drawn to animals "like moths to a porch light," as Wilson says. They offer a way to experience the physical and the social world. What is alive and what is not? What is human and what is not? Stuffed animals are soft but this thing is soft and responds to touch. I look my mother in the eye the same way I look this thing in the eye, but not this stuffed thing. When I move toward this thing, it *moves* away. I move, and it moves again. The spontaneity of the interaction keeps attracting the children to try and try again in a way that no television program, video game, or plastic toy ever could.

Perhaps Wilson is right that our affinity for animals is innate, but our culture also programs this reaction. From the time they are old enough to follow a story, the protagonists of children's books are, more often than not, animals. They see animals as heroes on television, in cartoons and video games, as toys and in movies. Children ages three to six report that 61 percent of their dreams feature animals, a percentage that drops dramatically as they age. By nine the figure is 36 percent, by fourteen the percentage has dropped to 20 and finally stabilizes at 7 percent. Of the first fifty words a child uses, seven of them are words for animals. In fact, "dog" and "cat" rank right up there with "mommy" and "daddy" in children's first vocabulary, and in many cases are more memorable to them than the words "juice," "milk," and "ball." Animals dominate a child's thinking, conscious and subconscious.

Researchers Aline and Robert Kidd observed six- to thirty-month-old children interacting with a battery-operated dog or cat, as well as their own dogs and cats. The Kidds found that the children made more noises and held and followed around the live animals much more than they did the toys. When researchers observed nine-month-old babies and their mothers left in a room first with an unfamiliar woman, then a dwarf rabbit, and later an animated wooden turtle, the children by far preferred the rabbit. In fact, they preferred the rabbit to their mothers, crawling around the room after it, trying to get a handful. The natural attractiveness of the interaction with animals also pays off in the mental development of the very young. Robert Poresky, human development and family studies professor at Kansas State University, questioned eighty-eight preschool children and their families from five midwestern daycare centers to establish how having pets influenced the development of young children. Children from families who owned pets, he found, scored higher in cognitive, social, and motor development.

Beyond the pure sensory stimulus animals provide, the other gift a well-domesticated pet brings to young children is an enhanced sense of security. Children trust the world to provide them food, warmth, and affection. While they can't get the first need met by an animal companion, the consistency of response they receive from pets can add to the children's expectation that they will be loved and valued. We develop a positive sense of self—our identity—from interactions that make us feel recognized, accepted, and admired; and from experiences that demonstrate what we do and how we feel is noticed. Pets offer all that in an unrestricted time frame. Parents can be too distracted by the hectic realities of day-to-day life to give their children as much reassurance as they need, but a pet will always listen to them and always has time to play.

Children form powerful attachments to their pets, which in many cases can be as strong as the attachment they feel toward a parent. They refer to their pets as members of the family. Preschool children believe that the animals listen to them, understand them, and in some cases the children are certain that the animals are communicating their feelings. In fact, studies show that even children as young as three believed that the love they feel for their pets is reciprocal. In one study, when elementary school-age children ranked their most significant relationships, pets got the highest scores as those most likely to be there "no matter what." A study of third graders asked to name their top-five relationships included their dogs as often as their mothers and fathers, and noted that they considered the animals more comforting when they were scared or ill than a best friend. A study of children in a war-torn region of Croatia found that pet-owning children had the lowest levels of post-traumatic stress disorder.

When I was a young boy, my parents got a toy Manchester terrier who definitely contributed to my overall development. Talk about similarity and difference! He was an amalgam of parts of the now-extinct black-and-tan terrier, the whippet, and West Highland white terrier. He was about the size of a Chihuahua, but in body type he looked like "Honey I Shrunk the Doberman Pinscher." We called him Skeeter because, in relation to the other farm animals and dogs, he was the size of a mosquito and he always seemed to be buzzing around. Originally bred for the dual purpose of chasing rabbits and killing rats, Manchester terriers lost a lot of their quick temper and snappiness when they lost their job as "verminators," but retained a lively spirit and alertness that fit in perfectly at our chaotic house.

Of all the animals on the farm, Skeeter was the first one who chose me. Skeeter followed me when the family scattered to opposite ends of the house or outside on our various chores. The preferred status that that conferred on me, at least in my own mind, was incredibly high. He probably chose me not for my sterling character or charisma, but because I frequently dropped a choice piece of meat from the dinner table into my cuffs for him to sniff out and snag. Or maybe it was because I let him sleep deep in my bed.

As winter crept up on the farm that first year we got Skeeter, my dad decided that he could sleep inside. In retrospect, the lack of discussion about this enormous change in the way we treated animals astounds me, but really it was the only humane choice. Winters on the edge of the vast southern Idaho desert are harsh and windy. Our coal furnace didn't put out much heat, and we compensated for that by pushing straw bales against the house's foundation and covering the windows with plastic to deflect the wind. Skeeter, who weighed ten pounds on a full stomach, would have had a hard time surviving the frost.

At night, Skeeter would take a running leap at my bed and dive underneath the covers, burrowing with his nose clear down my length until he came to a rest in the fold of my body—my very own fur-covered hot water bottle. Quite an advantage in the winter, but awfully hot during the summers. Overall, I was much more concerned about his comfort than I was about mine. There was always a sweet spot in the bed, a place where the temperature was pretty close to perfect. That was his spot. If he was shivering, no matter how hot I might be at that moment, I'd shut the window and pull the covers up around us. Later at night, when he was too hot, he would root up my side and join me cheek-to-cheek at the pillow. Even though he never demanded a thing, I set aside part of my spending money for gifts for the dog: a bright nylon collar and shiny ID tag, rainbow-colored Milk Bone dog biscuits, and silly little squeaky plastic things that only lasted a few days in his teeth. It gave me such pride to be able to give small tokens of what he so abundantly had given to me.

Children are the recipients of care, guidance, and protection but rarely have a chance to provide it, unless they have an animal for which they are responsible. Yet the next big transition in a young person's development comes when they start depending less on their parents and, through their own efforts, achieve a sense of mastery. Around 99 percent of children from the ages of three to thirteen say they want a pet. That doesn't mean that 99 percent of these children want the unpleasant secondary tasks of picking up dog poop or changing the litter box, but they're not getting the full benefit children can from the Bond if they don't.

When researchers examine the relationship between children and pets, they try to determine how attached the child is to the animal. One of the most popular measurement tools is the Companion Animal Bonding Scale, developed by Robert Poresky. The test asks, on a scale of always to never, how responsible the child is for the pet. Does he feed and clean up after it? How often does he stroke or pet the animal and how often does it sleep in his room? Other questions allow the child to rate the closeness of the relationship.

In Poresky's study of preschool children, the higher the children scored on the animal bonding scale, the higher their scores were in all measures of development and empathy. And when parents were asked to rate their child's social skills, those with high CABS scores also scored the highest on their ability to reassure and the lowest on being uncooperative. Clearly, the more general contact the child has with the pet, the more closely the child feels the Bond. If the child also takes on the responsibility of caring for the pet, the Bond becomes even stronger.

When children describe their relationships with their pets, they talk in terms of how they care for them and their routines. In this way, said Boris Levinson, a pioneer in the use of animals in psychotherapy, closeness to animals promotes self-esteem, self-control, and autonomy. The act of nurturing—meaning to nourish, educate, or train as well as to help grow—requires kids to read nonverbal signals and attend to them consistently. Through this, pets encourage kids to feel competent in far more complex ways than does learning to use the potty, eating their vegetables, or tying their shoes. Part of the constancy they provide, says UC Davis Applied Behavioral Science Prof. Brenda Bryant, is that their routine and needs remain constant while the world around the child makes increasingly more complex demands.

"Animals provide feedback to the kids, and the signals are very clear," Poresky said when we spoke about his research. "The dog sits on my foot and leans against me when he wants a walk. The realization that there is a creature who has feelings different than theirs takes them out of their egocentric point of view. Understanding this difference is a foundation of personality development. If you want your kids to be social creatures, they've got to develop empathy."

Children's interest in pets is the one strong element of childhood that survives as they mature, creating a constant in a changing world. In studying how animals and children nurture each other, Prof. Gail Melson asked parents to rate the way children in preschool, second grade, and fifth grade spent their time. As preschoolers, parents' estimates showed that children started off very connected to the life of the household. They scored high in playing with and caring for the pets, the elderly, and a younger sibling. Knowing the skill level of most preschoolers, I assume this figure really reflects the fact that they spend a lot of time with their mom, who calls upon them to help out, within their limitations. As they entered school and the pastimes of preschool fell away, the time caring for and playing with a pet increased. Their interest and concern for babies in general and their siblings in particular dropped, but the interest in their pets held steady, even as their chores with them increased.

What pets offer to parents is a "teachable moment," an experience that involves emotions, responsibilities, and consequences. There's a lot of popular lip service about teaching kids more responsibility. You can lecture your children all you want about proper behavior and good judgment, but the only time the words make sense to them is in the context of their actions. If they've received a poor mark at school, been caught in a lie, or let somebody down, they see and feel the results of what they've done or failed to do. These lessons can last a lifetime, but they don't come across as positive experiences, as the lessons from pets usually do.

Trying to get children to clean their rooms or spruce up the front yard can become a power struggle for the adult, and a child's deft exercise in trying to get out of responsibilities. What's the ultimate consequence of not cleaning your room? A dirty room and some sharp words from the parents. Yet unlike other household chores, pets respond. The consequence of not tending to the pet as you're expected to could cause that animal significant harm.

Mikkel and Lex have learned that feeding and watering the dogs, cats, and horses is a priority. Sometimes that means putting off logging onto the Internet to check e-mail or calling a friend. The act of feeding and caring for a pet—putting another's needs before yourself—is a lesson that should be learned early on. Such vital childhood competence deepens their Bond and, as a result, their emotional interdependence. The child and the pet form between them their own world of secrets that will never be betrayed, and long sessions of play where no one has something else on their minds. When it works, it can be a huge source of children's emotional stability and self-confidence, and the foundation of a more mature character. In studies in Japan and Australia, teachers reported higher levels of leadership and altruism in children who were the most familiar with animals.

Children who knew enough about their pets to describe their routine and behavior generally ranked themselves higher in competence. The parents of kindergarten children who were very attached to their pets reported fewer behavior problems, and their teachers had an easier time with them in class. In another study, children who said they received substantial emotional support from their pets were rated by their parents to be less anxious and withdrawn. Parents who want to encourage self-reliance in their children would do well to acquire a cat. A Swiss study of 540 children ages four, six, and eight noted that children who cared for cats scored higher on measures of self-reliance, and cat and dog owners both got higher marks on prosocial behavior.

Pets represent a teachable moment for the parents, too. When a married couple expresses doubts about their ability to raise children, child psychologist Foster Cline recommends an intriguing trial run. He suggests they borrow a friend's pet and see how well they can control it. The elements of raising a well-behaved pet are the same as those that should be used to discipline children. Parents of four- and two-legged children need to be firm, fair, and consistent. Yet parents give orders to their children that come across with undertones of an apology.

In my experience as a family veterinarian, I've found that when a family brings in an out-of-control pet, you can pretty much bet that their children have discipline problems, too. Cline says it's hard to determine if the effect of pets in encouraging responsible behavior is caused by pets, or if it simply takes place in families where the parents are already the kind of people who would foster responsibility. In some sense, it doesn't matter. The pets present an opportunity for the parents as well as the children to learn how to set standards, behave consistently, and give rewards for good behavior. Pets, like children, flourish on routine. They feel best when the adult is the alpha dog, completely in charge of making the arrangements.

Making the lines of authority clear is good for the development of children over the long term. Those who bond with animals from the ages of birth to five and later between the early adolescent ages of twelve to fifteen experience a long-term benefit from that relationship. Poresky found that people who had pets with whom they were especially close during those times of change later had a generally more positive sense of themselves, particularly adolescents. In a Swiss study of adolescents, pet owners reported a higher level of well-being and demonstrated less anxiety.

In his study of the similarities between the way humans and animals express emotions, Charles Darwin found many similarities between the way his infant son expressed fear and the way other species did: the same wide-open eyes and mouth, trembling muscles, rapid heartbeat, and hair standing on end. No wonder children raised around animals are better at understanding body language. Unlike the other, sometimes conflicting signals I got from members of my family, my dog Skeeter expressed love unconditionally. No matter what my report card looked like, how many points I'd scored in the game, if friends had been shuffled that day, or if I got a Mount Fuji–size pimple, Skeeter always greeted me as if my arrival home from school or in from the next room was the highlight of the day.

Besides that joyous validation, the other way that pets help a child's self-esteem is by being the envy of friends. There is nothing quite like the boost you can get from having a pet whom all of your friends wish was theirs. For instance, Luke, my Lab, was an incredible athlete, a beautiful, muscular dog just like a canine Worldwide Wrestling Federation star. Roughhousing that would have made a human friend furious delighted Luke, who was up for anything. I would tackle him from behind and kick legs out from under him and we'd tumble all over the ground. He was so strong that if I found a good-size stick, he would grab it between his jaws and allow me to swing him around like a helicopter for as long as I wanted.

Besides boosting my self-esteem, my brother Bobby's and my dogs also offered us emotional refuge. Dad's entire family suffered from manic depression, and he was not spared. Many days he was as warm, loving, and thoughtful a man as you'd ever want to meet, friend to all of the neighbor boys, our biggest fan at sporting events. But like Idaho weather, Dad could change moods in minutes. Sunny one minute, moving to overcast and dark, then erupting into a full storm, his voice cracking like thunder, lightning flashing from his eyes. On his highest high, he was like a rocket fueled by alcohol. He'd come home from the bar or stumble out of his hidden stash wanting to sell the farm, get a job in town, and buy a new car. Or his mood would take a sudden dip and he'd be crying or cussing and saying he wanted a divorce. "Let's split the sheets," he'd say to Mom. "I'll take the boys and you take the girls." Mom always maintained a sad yet stoic expression as she braced herself for the verbal blows that often came one after another until he fell asleep.

As a child, however, you don't understand a clinical diagnosis of manic depression or the result of drinking yourself senseless. You only understand that your smallest action, even an ill-timed glance, might set off a frightening rage. As my brother and I walked home across the fields from the afternoon school bus, we'd often make a game of trying to guess what kind of mood we'd find our father in when we got home. Sometimes we'd chant in a sweet sing-song voice that masked our real worry: "Daddy's in a huffy-puff! Daddy's in a huffy-puff!" My brother Bob and I would joke that Dad's hat rose hundreds of feet above his head to release the steam he generated as he walked around the farm.

Animals helped us here, too. Alan Entin, a Richmond, Virginia, psychologist who has studied the effects animals have on the family structure, talks about how the family pet can serve as a focus for emotions that family members don't feel safe expressing to one another. This can have a negative aspect, such as when the dad expresses a lot of affection for the family cat and much less for his wife and children. In my family, however, the incredible love, respect, and consideration my father demanded we give the animals served as a constant reminder of his better qualities.

My childhood chore for many years was harvesting the eggs from the fifty-odd chickens we kept. The job, as described to me by my father, was to reach up underneath that downy underside of each of the hens and extract the egg or eggs. To an antsy seven-year-old who wants to sit down to breakfast, this method seemed incredibly slow. One day I just threw my arms up and went "BLAH!" and they all roared off the nest boxes in a feather-flying panic. I walked the rows efficiently collecting my harvest, and was the first one done with chores and back in the house at the breakfast table. An excellent innovation, I thought, until the day Dad caught me. "This is not the way we do things 'round here," he said. "The better you take care of the animals, the better they take care of you." No matter how agitated my father became, no matter how violent or abusive, he never once took his anger out on the animals. He loved them and they loved him. All of them.

Bobby and I made it through some few dark summers on the farm side by side as we cared for the animals. They were dark because Dad was in such a deep depression, seldom leaving the house, while Bobby and I—sometimes with the help of a special few neighbors—took care of the entire farm, including planting, cultivating, and harvesting the crops, watering, milking the cows, taking care of the other livestock, everything. In these hard times, our glimmer of hope was Skeeter. My father loved that dog, and even in the depths of his darkest moods, Skeeter had a place of honor. Every night before dinner, Skeeter would get up on the chair and start to pray—with his head between his paws, doggie devotion mixed with doggie breath came steaming and streaming from his mouth. My dad would stand beside the dinner table cheering him on, saying: "Get down on it, Skeeter! Get down on it!" Later on at night when we would nestle together in the bed, I'd stroke my little pal, my very best friend, and tell him I knew he was the smartest, fastest, and most handsome dog of all, and everything was going to be all right. Everything was going to be just fine. It's only now that I realize that my telling it to Skeeter was a way of telling it to myself.

Children the world over turn to their pets in times of emotional stress. When they are feeling sad, the majority of German fourth graders surveyed turned to their animals, whom they said they preferred to the company of other children. A 1985 survey of Michigan children ages ten to fourteen established that 75 percent turned to their pets when they felt upset. Children gave animals high scores for their ability to listen, reassure, show appreciation, and provide companionship.

Nonanimal lovers think it's hilarious that we pet fanatics believe animals understand our emotions. I believe the same skills that allow a pet to detect the blur of a distant squirrel, the smell of a pheasant hiding in the weeds, the sound of the pizza delivery man before the doorbell rings, give them the ability to detect subtle shifts in one's moods, emotions, and needs.

When we first moved to Bonners Ferry, it was a time of transition for all of us, but most poignantly for our daughter Mikkel. She was approaching puberty and carrying the burden of those extra few pounds of baby fat, along with a severe case of shyness. Teresa and I would pick her up every day from this new school where she had few friends and she'd go directly to her room with her dog Scooter, who was her only refuge. I'd hear her in there talking steadily to the dog, explaining all of it down to the smallest detail. When she looks back on it with five years' distance, she is certain that Scooter understood her. "She didn't understand the words, of course," Mikkel says. "But she understood all the emotions."

My childhood situation with my father seems extreme, but emotional turmoil is commonplace in the lives of many children these days. The pressures kids face have escalated exponentially in the last two decades. A study of modern childhood by the American Institute of Stress said teen suicide and homicide rates have tripled, childhood obesity has jumped 50 percent, and more children are living at the poverty level now than twenty years ago. Now it's not unusual for teachers to see anxiety attacks in nine-year-olds, and stress-related ulcers before age twelve. As a result, elementary schools have started offering stress-reduction classes that involve meditation and visual imagery.

The American family isn't what it used to be. The *Leave It to Beaver/ Father Knows Best* model with parents who stayed married and a mom who didn't work outside the home was more the rule back in the 1950s when I was growing up. Such families are rare now. According to the 2000 Census, just 23.5 percent of households are now "traditional" families. Meanwhile, other percentages are up: families headed by single mothers or fathers, people living alone, and unmarried couples. The number of families headed by single mothers has increased by 25 percent in the last ten years. More than half of all whites and 75 percent of all African Americans will spend some part of their childhood in a single-parent household. As Prof. Gail Melson points out in her fascinating book on animals and children, *Why the Wild Things Are*, these demographic trends show that children are more likely to grow up in a home with a pet than they are in one that has two parents.

Dr. Wilfried Goecke, a veterinarian friend of mine from Denmark, told me that when famed Danish company Lego was starting a new line called Lego Villages, they asked Danish children to write down who they thought should be in the village. Lego was shocked to find out that people said, "Mom, brother or sister, and pets." When they asked what happened to Dad, the children said, "We play with Mom, our brothers and sisters, and especially with our pets. Dad's never around for us to play with."

Mothers who work outside the home, whether they are single moms or married, see pets as a way to normalize those lonely hours a child may spend at home after school. Not only are employed mothers more likely to acquire pets, but the more hours they are employed, the more time the child spends caring for the pet and hence the increased closeness and importance of the Bond. In fact, another study of seven- and ten-year-olds whose mothers worked showed that the children of working moms were more likely to describe their pets as special friends.

The studies point to how important a pet can be for the whole family that surrounds a latchkey kid. When both parents work outside the home, the world becomes smaller. The children are less likely to be involved with friends, youth groups, and other activities. The exhausted parents have less inclination to enlarge their world too, making the pet an important catalyst for spontaneity and play in the household.

When Fred Seford's mother left the family before he reached the age of one, his father's four dogs "became his brothers and sisters," says his father, John. Raised in a family that bred Labradors, John owned three, and a one-hundred-forty-five-pound malamute. Despite the size of these dogs, John had them so well trained that by the age of three, thirty-five-pound Fred could walk all four of them and get them to stop just by raising his hand.

As a single-parent family, John and Fred moved around from one leased home to another until they bought a place of their own near Pikes Peak in Colorado. By this time Fred was eleven years old, the other dogs had died and, John thought, his son was old enough to care for a dog of his own. Fred pored over the specifications of different breeds, with a fondness for the larger ones that had been his siblings when he was a toddler. He'd pretty much settled on getting a Newfoundland when a friend told the Sefords that St. Bernards were more of a one-person dog. Fred wanted a dog that would be his and his alone. He finally decided to get a female St. Bernard puppy he named Domino.

John, like many parents, thought his son would benefit by having another creature rely on him. He was pleased at how quickly Fred adjusted to the routine of caring for Domino. John also benefited by how Domino helped to assuage some of the single-parent guilt. "He's a single child. I wanted Domino to take away some of the loneliness."

John often works from home. On the days he has to go to the office, Fred used to go to an afterschool program. Now that he's older, he has the choice to come home to Domino, the ultimate playmate. "Domino is always ready, all the time excited," John said. When she was more of a puppy, she'd run alongside Fred on his skateboard or bound ahead as they hiked. Now that she's six months old (and eighty-five pounds!), she's more coordinated. Fred tries out his passing arm and Domino retrieves the football.

John wasn't anticipating how much the dog would enhance the sense that three makes a family. She's a great playmate, but she's also a watchful mom. Fred and Domino have a snack together when he gets home from school, and she sits patiently while he does his homework before they go out to play. She sits outside the bathroom door listening to him brush his teeth, and at night sits beside him until he completes his bath. Although Domino is definitely Fred's dog, she likes her time with John. At night, all three of them tuck Fred into bed and Domino, who likes to stay up a little later, tags around after John. Around ten o'clock she gives the house a thorough sniff to make sure everything is where it should be, and spends the rest of the night on Fred's bed or next to it. Combined, all of Domino's habits have served to take some of the pressure off John. "Instead of coming in and being the entertainment, I get to come in and just be Dad," John says. "It's much better for both of us having her around."

John hasn't yet come up against the rough times of adolescence, but it's not too far away. For Dee Parr, a mom whose daughter, Christine, is a sixth grader at my son's school in Bonners Ferry, animals have become a way for mother and daughter to keep communicating even when other issues have become too heated to discuss. Christine has always been the kind of person animals are drawn to. People often comment that a cat who won't go to strangers, or a dog who always growls, reacts calmly to Christine. For Christine's part, she craves contact with animals, and so does her mom. At night after Dee gets off work, they have a job gentling foals and young mules. They stroke and handle young mules and horses to desensitize them to human touch, which makes them easier to handle and train when they mature. Both mother and daughter look forward to going to work. For Dee, it's a great stress reducer, and an activity about which they have no conflict. "We're starting to fight a lot at this age, and I'm scared that I might start losing control and be unable to reach her. I think it is important to try to find some kind of common ground," Dee says. "On a certain level, we communicate better because of this."

I've seen the bridge a mutual love of animals can build between sparring parents and children in my own home. A few years back, it seemed like Teresa and Mikkel were fighting about the smallest and most insignificant things. As Mikkel later explained, she'd realized that her mom is a pushover. Certainly one of the things I value the most in my wife is her compassion and sensitivity; her exquisite ability to respond to the needs of others. To an adolescent, this can make an adult an easy figure to manipulate. Mikkel realized that if she just got mad enough or hurt enough, Teresa would give in. Eventually Mikkel stopped respecting her, and every situation became a fractious test of limits, a painful power play.

Last year, Teresa and I decided to give in to Mikkel's endless requests to get a show horse of her own. She'd become interested in western pleasure riding, a competitive exhibition of horsemanship. Teresa is an experienced horsewoman with a keen eye for value in horses, and the two of them spent hours in front of the VCR looking at tapes of prospective horses for Mikkel. They even flew as far as Alabama to review candidates, but settled on one quite close to home.

When we got Glo Lopin, of course there were an endless number of decisions to be made about where to board her, who would coach Mikkel, what kind of outfit she should compete in. Now when the catalogs arrive from the horse companies, my daughter and her mother squeal as they review the different looks and accessories. They spend many hours together en route to competitions and discuss everything from school and boys to the politics of the horse world. Mikkel, like Teresa, is shy but competitive. They have begun to see their similarities both in the way they view the world and their interaction with it, especially when Mikkel took first place in her first competition. Their arguments have dwindled from three a day to maybe one a week. "My mom really knows a lot about horses," Mikkel said. "I definitely respect her opinion."

That vital link to a pet, besides increasing a child's sense of competence and general notion that they are a fair and reliable person, can also have a small but positive impact on intelligence. Poresky surveyed eighty-eight Kansas children and found those with higher scores on his companion animal bonding scale also scored, on average, five points higher in IQ. Although some, including Poresky, tend to think that this number statistically isn't that significant, he also said that he believes if he'd had a larger sample of children the percentage of increase very likely would have been higher. He doesn't want to give all the credit to the pet, however. Mirroring Foster Cline's question about whether the pet is the cause or just one of a number of positive factors in a responsibly run household, Poresky said, "The overall quality of the home environment is a much more important factor in a child's intellectual development than the impact of the interaction with a pet."

In Salt Lake City, pets have become the bridge to a very specific positive intellectual development. For the last two years, trained teams of dogs and humans have helped kids who have trouble reading to jump whole grade levels in just a few months in a simple program where children read to dogs.

The brainchild of Intermountain Therapy Animals member Sandi Martin, the program started in 1999 in one of the most culturally diverse elementary schools in the city, Lynn M. Bennion Elementary. Although reading specialist Kris Andreasen was skeptical that the program would work, she decided the school had nothing to lose from the experiment, and asked teachers to recommend some of their students who were having the most difficulties. When Sandi and her Portuguese water dog, Olivia, arrived with Kathy McNulty and her akita, Kyoshi, they found a representation of the American melting pot. All of the students had English as their second language, and each one of them was from a different country: Mexico, Somalia, Bosnia, China, Korea, Japan, Tibet, and Iraq. The one language they all spoke was dog.

Kathy had trained grave, dignified Kyoshi to pay attention to the book by hiding razor-thin slivers of treats at random intervals among the pages. As a result of this expectation, Kyoshi stares as if the most fascinating story ever told were unfolding before his snout, and the book holds his interest even if the child stumbles over a word. Kathy and Sandi gently encourage the children by suggesting that the word the child has just stumbled over is one the dog doesn't know the meaning of. The child then defines the word or asks for an explanation.

The afternoon I observed the two teams and the children, I could see how much affection and stimulation the children were getting from the dogs. Sandi said she hadn't anticipated when they began working at Bennion that the children who were reading challenged would also be socially challenged. Many of them had few friends, and their lack of success at school made them more withdrawn and therefore more isolated. But working with the dogs helped them in the social arena, as well.

The children each get twenty minutes with the dog: roughly two minutes to greet the dog, fifteen minutes of reading, and a few more minutes at the end to say good-bye. It was clear how emotionally dependent the children were on the dogs. They chose books whose themes, they assured Sandi and Kathy, would appeal to the dogs. They leaned into the dogs and their companions as the session progressed, completely relaxed and comfortable. It looks sweet and it feels good, but it also gets results. The first six children they worked with showed marked improvement in just ten weeks. Four of them improved their reading scores a full grade level, and the other two jumped by two grade levels. The school has over one hundred tutors working with this reading-challenged population, but the happiest and most successful students are those working with the dogs.

This program offers undivided and nonjudgmental attention from another adult and the dog. The other aspect of the program that Sandi didn't expect is that it conferred status on the children. As she and Kathy walk into the school on Wednesday afternoons against the tide of students on their way home, many of the kids beg to be included in the program.

"This isn't for the kind of person who likes structure, because each child presents a different challenge," said Kathy. "And you've got to be able to think on your feet." She described her Buddha-like dog Kyoshi's approach to life as "start slow and taper off." One afternoon a little boy who is especially enamored of Kyoshi had chosen an adventure story that featured a dog. In the middle of a dramatic scene, Kyoshi slumped against Kathy and drifted off to sleep. Kathy was nimble in her explanation. She told the boy that he was reading so well and the scene was so interesting that Kyoshi had closed his eyes so he could envision it more completely.

On the day of our visit, Josh, a wiry third grader, was having a hard time settling down to read. He chose *The Silly Goose* by Dav Pilkey, a humorous book about the adventures of cartoonish geese that had more pictures than text. Although Josh had jumped a full grade level in his reading scores in the previous six weeks, you couldn't see any improvement at first. Josh is from a fractured family that doesn't place a high value on education. Josh wriggled and squirmed, pretty much ignoring Olivia after a hello pat on the head, and tried to skip pages in the story. "I think you need to sit a little closer," said Sandi, "Olivia is straining to see the pictures." As he moved closer, he started to stroke Olivia, who leaned on him for the touch. The pressure of her body alongside his relaxed him, and by the time their session was coming to an end, he was leaning up against Sandi, too, reading without distraction. "So you think if you read with Olivia long enough she'll learn how to read it herself?" I asked. Josh looked at me as if I were one in a long series of stupid adults. "She can't read!" he said with exasperation, then added proudly, "She needs me to read to her."

While most reading specialists find the approach unconventional, a lot of different aspects of successful reading approaches are coordinated through the dogs. Studies, most notably by Johns Hopkins Professor James Lynch, prove that children's blood pressure drops and they relax while reading to a friendly dog. Reading experts say that children who are placed regularly in the presence of books become better readers, particularly if they can be made to see that reading is fun.

The program has been so successful that Salt Lake City's main public library established "Dog Day Afternoons," a reading program with dogs in the children's library on Saturday afternoons where children receive bone-shaped bookmarks. Now the program is in every branch library in Salt Lake and is being expanded in the public schools. Sandi has consulted with libraries in Louisiana, Missouri, and California.

A month after I visited Bennion Elementary, Olivia, who was only three years old, was suddenly stricken with aggressive cancer. For the two weeks she lived after diagnosis, doctors gave her something for the pain and something to stimulate her appetite. After a series of elaborate meals hand-prepared by Sandi, Olivia died in Sandi's arms at the veterinarian office.

Sandi is trained as a grief counselor and knew not to try to hide the truth from the kids with some mysterious euphemism. Frequently parents want to shield their children from the pain of knowing their pet has died, mainly because the parents are afraid of their own feelings and don't want to appear to lose control in front of the kids. If you as a family don't grieve this loss, you are robbed of a chance to honor that relationship. The family that doesn't allow the child to experience the death of a beloved pet is also missing another benefit of the Bond to children: a forum for them to experience the life cycle, from birth to aging to death.

Sandi was once lecturing about grieving with children to a large audience of adults. She was stopped by the sound of a sob from the back of the room. She asked the fifty-year-old woman if she'd like to share what she was feeling. She said that when she was six, her parents had had to euthanize her dog, and they explained his absence by saying he'd run away. For years, she'd thought that her dog just didn't love her anymore.

"Say you tell the kids, I gave the dog away," said Carolyn Butler, coordinator of Changes, a program at the vet school at Colorado State University that helps families deal with the stress of pet loss and serious illness. "Then the child will want to know if the new owner is a man or a woman. Does he live around here? Could we ever go visit? Could he send us a picture? Pretty soon, you're six lies in. Later, when you decide the child is emotionally ready to handle it, you tell the truth. Then they start to wonder what else you've lied about."

When I was first practicing as a veterinarian, the procedure was to take the animal to the back room out of the sight and touch of the human companion, inject the lethal solution, and bring the body back in a plain cardboard box. Standard procedure, too, was not to allow humans to see their animals when they were being treated or hospitalized. When I got my own practice, I encouraged the human companions to visit their sick four-legged children. If you accept the studies that say humans definitely think of their pets as family members, people would never stand for the hospital banning them from visiting. They'd tear the walls down to get to their sick family member. I also found that the pets recovered more quickly if they saw their "parents" daily, and it was easier on the human family, too. Gradually this influenced the way we handled euthanizing a pet. I wanted the families included, and I was always impressed by how appropriately the children behaved.

The Changes program has outfitted a room for the family to go to when their dog is going to pass on. It has subdued lighting, a soft mat on the floor, blinds on the windows, and benches at one corner that look like small-scale church pews. There are compartments under the bench seats that hold condolence cards, bags, and small scissors so the family can capture a lock of their pet's hair and clay slugs into which they can make a paw imprint (like a permanent fingerprint). "People need linking objects," says Laurel Lagoni, Changes's managing director, "something to link them to their animal as they go through their grief."

Parents frequently call for advice on whether or not to tell the children. Carolyn Butler remembered one family whose golden retriever had died and the kids were asking to see it, but the parents were too scared to show them their fallen friend. Carolyn persuaded them to bring the children in, even though one was under the age of five. The animal was carefully groomed, her coat brushed out soft and silky, but the parents were still scared. They didn't even want to enter the room. The kids led the way. They went in and laid their hands on the dog very softly and looked silently for a while. The littlest one turned back to Mom and Dad to comfort them. "It's okay," she said. "She's just cold like she came in from the snow." Carolyn and Laurel were not surprised. "Start by trust-ing the children," Carolyn said. "They always know what they need. Parents learn to respect their children when they see how they handle death."

Olivia and Sandi missed the reading program the week before Olivia died. By the time Josh came for his session, he'd already heard about Olivia's illness. He came in striking out, using foul language, and trying to agitate a few of the other kids. Lance, one of the reading specialists, asked Josh if he wanted to talk about Olivia. Josh said he didn't want to talk about it. He didn't really care. Lance persisted. He said he needed to talk to someone about how sad he was feeling, and he was hoping to speak to Josh because he knew how close Olivia and he had been. Josh sat down to comfort Lance and fifteen minutes later he was sobbing in Lance's lap.

We're always talking about raising self-esteem in children, but what really needs raising is the *family's* esteem, its perception of itself as a unit of people with a shared set of humane values, common goals, and a multitude of ways to nurture one another. In the hectic times in which we live, these values and goals can fall from view as we concentrate on what we lack as a family and a society, instead of on what we give to one another. This is where the Bond can play a vital role in the family. Each of us feels a vital connection to the animals through which we can demonstrate our best selves, our highest values, and, with practice, learn to nurture those abilities in our treatment of other family members and as citizens of the world. But failing that, as in the case of my family and my father, a pet can serve as an emotional refuge, a patient listener, and a connective tissue that gives the family, no matter its trials, a sense of purpose and belonging.

Untying the Knot of a Troubled Childhood

THERE IS PERHAPS NO MORE powerful image of childhood gone horribly wrong than the sight of hundreds of teenagers fleeing Columbine High School while two of their classmates murdered thirteen and injured twenty-one children. Our schools are supposed to be safe, the classroom secure from all but the petty sniping of cliques and jilted sweethearts. And our kids are not supposed to be planting bombs or packing shotguns, as Eric Harris and Dylan Klebold did that day. Parents are supposed to be loving and consistent, too, but it doesn't always work out that way. In trying to reach children whom society has traumatized or abandoned, therapists, as they did in working with the traumatized survivors of Columbine, increasingly use animals to break through their defenses so they can start to heal.

Most of us watched our televisions in horror in April 1999 as over and over again we saw those signature pieces of video footage: children running from Columbine High School as shots rang out behind them and one falling limp, headfirst, from a second story window. For us, it was a tragedy we were able to turn off, but not so for the people of Littleton, Colorado. The signs of posttraumatic stress were all over town for months afterward, from the escalation in shoot-'em-up playacting among young children to adults and children who had trouble concentrating.

Most stricken were the Columbine High School students, some of whom were so terrorized they literally ran out of their shoes on the day of the shootings and were found three miles from the school with bloody, raw feet. For months afterward, they felt the trauma in their minds and their bodies in the form of tingling in the feet of those who had run so far so fast, and back trouble in those who had fled the building fearing that they were about to be shot in the back.

When school began again, many formerly stellar students' grades dropped, friendships dissolved, and substance abuse skyrocketed, as did angry outbursts. Despite the fact that the school district had blocked off the library where the shootings took place, students saw traumatic reminders of that day everywhere, which tripped their nervous systems, making them hypervigilant. Some of the kids' memories of trauma were tripped by the sight of pizza. Harris and Klebold had scattered ninety-five bombs around the school, many of them in the cafeteria, where a large portion of the school's two thousand students would be getting their lunch at 11:20, the moment the bombs were timed to explode. When they didn't go off, Harris and Klebold started shooting at them, triggering the sprinkler system, which flooded the room. Those trapped in the cafeteria remembered the sight of pizza floating by.

"Columbine was a kid-on-kid tragedy," said Marguerite McCormack, project director at Columbine Connections Resource Center, a place where people traumatized by the event could receive free counseling. "These were kids who saw horrendous things. Intrapersonal trauma is the worst kind to recover from. But trauma is highly treatable."

One little boy had been waiting with his mother in a car at a traffic light when terrified students covered in blood and broken glass ran past them. After that, he would not talk, a sign of posttraumatic stress syndrome. After a severe emotional shock, the left side of the brain, the part that controls verbal skills, shuts down. "This child was all locked up. He couldn't move forward, couldn't sleep, couldn't eat," Marguerite said.

Fortunately, Columbine Connections was crawling with friendly animals. Marguerite said she was simply lucky that the therapists she hired were animal crazy, because she'd never planned to try to reach her clients through pets. One clinician had asked if she could bring her English bulldog puppy to work, and Marguerite agreed. The next time the little boy came in, he gravitated to the puppy. The staff was so pleased that he had found something he could respond to that Marguerite encouraged all of her staff to bring in their pets.

The clinicians began to ask if their clients had animals and, if so, they tried to get them to spend more time with them. One client was a thirteen-year-old girl who had watched two kids being shot outside the cafeteria window. After the shooting, many of her friendships had disintegrated, and she was having trouble sleeping and eating. She, like many other students, was also having trouble concentrating in school. "It's not that she wasn't trying," Marguerite said. "She was failing because she couldn't remember."

Trauma affects brain chemistry in a number of ways, Marguerite explained. It suppresses the manufacture of serotonin, the neurochemical that influences sleep, depression, memory, mood stabilization, and impulse control. The net result is that traumatized people don't have the capacity to soothe or reward themselves. Another neurological phenomenon that makes treating traumatized clients tough is that trauma lodges itself in a part of the brain that is not immediately accessible to rational thought. Columbine Connections clients couldn't be argued into forgetting what had happened. No cheerful suggestions that "this too shall pass" made any sense to them. What they needed was a way to connect to the world.

The clinicians saw how much joy the girl got from playing with the dogs at the clinic, and they encouraged her to spend more time with her own dogs. Over the course of several visits, the girl said she'd started lying with her dogs on the couch and using one as a pillow when she slept. She got better in part because she was able to make this connection, Marguerite says.

Counselors also used animals to reach the children after Kip Kinkel killed two of his fellow students and wounded twenty-five at Thurston High School, in a small community just outside Springfield, Oregon; Cindy Ehlers and her dog, Bear, were part of the therapy team that conducted group sessions with the traumatized students. The National Organization for Victim Assistance, specially trained trauma counselors, were flown in from Washington, D.C., to work with the children, but were having a difficult time getting the kids to express themselves.

The students' reactions were all over the place. One girl, who had been shot in the back and was confined to a wheelchair, made constant jokes. Most of the boys didn't want to talk about their feelings. Another girl was furious, and threatened to kill Kip Kinkel for taking away her innocence, if she ever got the chance. This girl had been hardened by the experience. She had started wearing thick makeup and provocative clothing.

When Cindy and Bear entered the first session, Bear was drawn to a girl who was slumped in her chair, withdrawn behind a curtain of hair across her face. Bear stood directly in front of her, but she didn't acknowledge Bear. Bear wiggled a little closer, then a little closer, and made a funny noise. Not a growl, but a noise of sympathy. The girl looked up and grabbed Bear and brought her into her lap. She held her close and as she did she began to sob openly, and then to describe what she was feeling.

From the boys, Cindy sensed incredible anger, but she didn't know how to help bring it out into the room. She decided that the boys could try to get Bear to do tricks, and divided them into teams, competing for obedience. Working with Bear became a metaphor for engaging with the world. Bear would not respond if they were rough with her or angry when she didn't obey them promptly. To get what they wanted from Bear, they had to handle their anger and communicate clearly.

By the day of the first anniversary of the shooting, the children in the therapy group had made remarkable progress. Many of the boys put Bear through her tricks without a single raised voice or sharp word. The girl who had affected the hard exterior had dropped her harsh makeup and started wearing more modest clothing, and generally the group had started to move through their anger and sorrow.

Thurston High had a ceremony to mark the anniversary of the horrible event. The kids wanted Cindy and Bear to attend, but they were refused by the administration, which was very strict about keeping the campus closed to outsiders. Cindy's feelings were bruised a bit, but she got over it. "Bear was a tool to get them to the point where they could start the healing process," Cindy said, noting that Bear became Delta's Service Dog of the Year in 1999. "Bear was like emotional search and rescue. Go in and bring the emotions out. Once she did that, it was okay if her job ended there."

It seems almost too simple, too tied up with a bow to say that the solution to life-shattering trauma is to spend time with a dog, but Marguerite McCormack of Columbine points to a very specific therapeutic benefit.

"Trauma does damage the ability to form a relationship," Marguerite said. "It destroys the belief in a safe universe. If you don't have a sense of trust or a sense of safety, how can you form a relationship? Animals are safe. This is a relationship that will not bring you harm. In the fold of this relationship with the animal, it is possible to develop a vision of a life where you are calm, people are nice, and the universe is in its right place."

Animals were one of a number of techniques that the clever, compassionate clinicians at Columbine Connections used to try to knit the survivors back together. "We used whatever we could. If a person had tremendous spiritual faith, we used that," Marguerite said. The lucky advent of animals was a positive focus of attention for both therapist and child that greatly speeded up recovery.

Sometimes it's difficult for a therapist to hold herself back just at the moment when a child is making a therapeutic breakthrough, because occasionally that moment puts both the animal and the patient at risk. Dr. Elaine Litton is a Vista, California, therapist whose German shepherd colleague, Cisco, is her cotherapist. One of Elaine's patients was a four-year-old girl who had been physically and emotionally abused by her father's girlfriend and one of her grandparents. She also had experienced the repeated loss of her mom, who would have her for a while, then lose her to foster care because she was unreliable, repeating the abuse and loss.

The child always wanted to see Cisco, but then would lose interest and get toys out. One day they had dolls out and the little girl started to talk very directly to the dolls about the physical abuse, saying, "I'm just a little girl." Elaine sensed that the emotional scab of this painful wound was coming off, giving her a chance to validate the girl's feelings. "This wasn't the right thing to do," Elaine offered. "This shouldn't have happened to you." The girl immediately set the dolls down, walked over to Cisco and straddled him like a pony, resting her head on the side of his neck and holding on so tight her knuckles were blanched.

Elaine watched uncomfortably, wondering if she should intervene. Even though he was well socialized, Cisco didn't like this kind of confinement. Would he snap for the first time? Cisco did not move a muscle;

he sensed both the little girl and Elaine needed him to just be there. The girl couldn't be physically close to Dr. Litton, but she could be to Cisco. There was a tremendous release of energy in the room. Elaine told the little girl after she let go that Cisco had never let anybody do that before. "You're a very special girl, and he just validated that," Elaine told her. That day was a dramatic breakthrough in the girl's treatment, after which Dr. Litton was more trusted and effective.

At residential facilities where children are recovering from a lifetime of abuse and neglect, animals can be a vital therapeutic tool that can serve as a catalyst for growth and change.

On the banks of the Hudson River sixty miles north of New York City is Green Chimneys, a 166-acre farm where some of the toughest kids in New York have been ordered by the court to live. Here their progress toward being integrated back into society is boosted by their relationships with farm animals.

Many of these kids have been sent to Green Chimneys because their parents were either unwilling or incapable of caring for them. Some have already run afoul of the law. They have grown up surrounded by violence, abuse, and neglect, and have witnessed and committed horrific crimes. Yet despite the fact that many have come from prison and psychiatric facilities, there are no bars or tall gates keeping them inside the rolling acres of Green Chimneys, a place that feels simultaneously like a family farm and a summer camp.

The facility is a former dairy farm, and many of the buildings have been converted from their original use to structures for staff and facilities for the one hundred residents and thirty day students. Beyond the charming new school building and residence hall, both constructed to look like barns, is an actual barn that houses some of the therapy assistants for the staff and the residents: the horses, sheep, pigs, chickens, cattle, and birds of prey.

The whole place was designed and created by founder Sam Ross who, at seventy-three, has more energy than a Jack Russell on espresso. When his dad purchased the farm in 1948, Sam wanted to establish a boarding school for girls and boys. He kept the animals because he believed they would be a great lure for kids who were raised, as he was, in the asphalt and concrete of New York City.

Therapists kept sending him children with emotional problems, and Sam found that his program of having them work daily with the farm animals helped them make rapid progress toward being more responsible and trusting.

"Children come here because they haven't made it in school. They haven't made it at home. They haven't made it in the community. They've been told they will never amount to anything," said Sam from his office, a glass-walled greenhouse that faces the sloping main lawn. He says that the secret to these kids' success really isn't much of a secret at all. "It's really very simple. You take a child who is having problems, who's shy, who's not mixing well, and suddenly you turn him loose with an animal, and they get megalick therapy."

Sam makes it sound as if you put a troubled kid in a horse stall, and pick him up a few months later cured. His charming phrase disguises the rigorous attention paid to the kids from the moment they walk through the white picket fence.

For the first month after a child arrives at Green Chimneys, he or she isn't allowed to interact with the animals. The staff watches closely for signs of an abusive past that might make it, at least initially, unsafe for the animals to be around the child. This careful monitoring is a part of everything the child does at Green Chimneys. At the end of each week, everyone on the staff who has regular contact with the child rates his or her status on a scale from one to five in several areas, including hygiene, peer relations, interactions with authority figures, academics, eye-hand coordination, and reality perception. In addition, social workers in New York City assess the home situation the child came from and might be returning to.

After a month of getting acclimated to the routine, the children are allowed to go up to the barn and work with Suz Brooks, a licensed therapist who supervises their interactions with the animals. When the kids have their first contact with animals, she is right alongside them, monitoring their behavior as a way of diagnosing their psychological state.

As Sam Ross asks, how do you reach a cynical eight-year-old? The paradox of Green Chimneys is that while the staff is childlike and joyful, the children are hardened.

"Most of our children haven't been touched very much, and certainly not in very good ways," said Suz. "And we aren't legally and ethically able to touch the children in the way that they really need. The animals provide that touch, that sense of nurturance. There's a lot of healing from a living being that doesn't try to move away, but is just with you."

On a day when Timothy, one of the students, had just found out his drug-addicted parents had surrendered their parental rights to him, he had sat by himself at recess and fallen asleep in class, Suz recalled. She hoped that the farm, and particularly a llama named Angel, would be a safe place for him to release his feelings and receive some affection back.

Timothy had a long history with Angel, who had been a parent of sorts for Tim. She had rightly earned her name for her calm, stoic nature. She would sit quietly chewing her cud as kids hugged her and poured out their hearts to her. Tim even called her "Momma" when they were together. He'd ask: "Hey, Momma, who loves you?"

Timothy sought Angel out. He found her sitting in the corral. He sat next to her and buried his face in her neck fur. Suz stood back at a respectful distance, knowing that this was a kid who didn't really know how to cry and had never had an adult to hold him. She waited and Timothy started to sob as he clung to Angel, letting out pain and years and years of sorrow. He sobbed for almost an hour, and Angel stayed with him munching stoically on her cud.

The scientific literature that supports the physiological changes that humans experience when they are in close contact with an animal certainly hints as to why Timothy could finally emote while he hugged Angel. The children of Green Chimneys are an anxious population whose life experiences have shown them time and again that no good can come out of exposing your vulnerability to another human being. With his arms around Angel, Timothy's blood pressure most likely dropped, his breathing began to regulate, and, no longer fighting the world in a hard shell of a body, he could release his feelings.

The flip side of this incredibly deep sorrow is intense rage. A lot of what Suz deals with is the appropriate expression of anger. When a child first comes to the farm, she gives the child small animals to hold, and watches the way they hold them and touch the larger ones. Their demeanor with the animals can be a starting off point for allowing them to see how their behavior affects all living creatures around them.

When children have trouble controlling their anger, Suz places them in close contact with Green Chimneys' donkeys because they are especially apprehensive around people. In order to get close to them, Suz says, a human has to project calm self-assurance. The donkeys' response to anger is so quick, they are an excellent source of feedback on how an aggressive young person behaves.

Suz carefully managed an interaction between the donkeys and Gil, a thirteen-year-old who had been at Green Chimneys for two years but who still was having difficulties making friends.

Suz placed Gil in the small donkey pen. His presence there caused the donkeys to group together at a corner with their ears pinned back. Gil said he wasn't afraid of the donkeys, so Suz suggested he take his hands out of his pockets and lift his head up to look at them. He did this quickly, as he did almost all his movements, and the donkeys stared uncomfortably as they shifted around. Gil looked defeated.

Suz asked him who he cared for, and Gil responded that he cared for his mom. When she asked him to try to describe where that caring feeling rested in his body, all Gil could do was shrug his shoulders. After some thought, he located the feeling in his heart and in his head. Suz asked him to stay in touch with that feeling as he looked at the donkeys. When she asked him if the donkeys liked having him in the pen, he said no. They looked as if they were unhappy, scared, and wanted him to go away, Gil said. Suz's therapeutic leap was to ask him if he believed other kids sometimes looked at him that way. Gil looked off into space, and the affirmative shake of his head was barely perceptible.

Here was a way to connect with him, Suz realized. He was examining his actions, not defending them. If she managed this episode carefully, he might make progress in picking up on social cues and understand the impact of his body language. Suz suggested that there was a way to approach the donkeys that would make them feel more comfortable. She asked him to try to generate that feeling of warmth for his mother as he approached the donkeys.

He stood for a minute or two, then reached out his hands as he approached the donkeys. Once he crossed into their safety zone, they backed away. As they backed away, he moved toward them until he was chasing them around the pen futilely. Suz told him to stop and try to understand why they were backing away, but Gil was confused. Suz imitated his movements, and the donkeys, whom Gil knew to be normally drawn to her, backed away as well.

"All I cared about was that I wanted to pet the donkeys," Suz explained to Gil. "I wasn't paying attention to what was going on for them; whether they wanted to be petted right at that moment. The intensity of that action scared them. Let's try it again."

Although Gil did not succeed that day, over time he did learn how to approach the donkeys, which taught him lessons in building trust and how to approach others in a nonthreatening manner. In time, Gil received the concrete rewards for learning this lesson. The donkeys came to vie for his touch, and gradually he moved this lesson out into the world of his peers.

One of the hardest populations to reach is children with autism. The sorrow of parents of such children is that they seem indifferent and unable to form any bonds. They are also tactilely defensive, meaning that they shrink from touch. Occupational therapist Mona Sams works with autistic children and llamas on sensory integration.

Autistic children are very sensitive in their hands, but not so in their feet. Mona starts off by rubbing their feet over the dense, woolly fur of one of her four llamas. Next she encourages them to bury their feet deep in the fur. Eventually, she stands them on top of the animals so they can feel the llama's spine, the contrast between soft and firm. She gradually works toward getting the kids to touch the llama with their hands. "It helps to integrate their senses," Mona says. "If you introduce this right, they begin to enjoy it."

A study under way at the People Pet Partnership at my alma mater, Washington State University, shows dogs can hold the attention of autistic children too. The study, conducted by François Martin and his staff, videotaped autistic children under three conditions: with a counselor and a ball, then a counselor with a stuffed animal, and lastly with a dog, in forty-five sessions over a span of fifteen weeks. The children watched the dog and talked about him more and for longer periods of time than they did the other two objects, preliminary results indicate.

I've watched some of the tapes, which François and his staff have very carefully coded in exhaustive hours of reviewing. What those figures miss is the dramatic change in energy of the children when the live dog is in the room. In one of the sessions I saw, the ball rolled away and the child sat impassively, as he did next to the plush toy. But with the dog, he was up and interacting. He was also a lot more cooperative. He followed instructions to brush the dog and when he and the therapist spoke, he used the plural pronoun "we." When the dog moved away, he moved after it.

This seems small, of course, but small steps are all these children can tolerate. Mona has one client who never thought she'd be able to hold a conversation with her son, as he seemed blank, with no interest in any form of communication. After two years working with Mona and her menagerie, he does speak and smile. Mona will not take all the credit for his progress, as he is in lots of other therapy, including speech. But she's happy to take credit for the spark that got things started.

Mona has a unique job. Each morning she loads a few of her llamas, her dogs, perhaps a pig, and some smaller, cuddlier animals such as rabbits and hamsters on to her stock trailer, which is decorated with the name "Mona's Ark." She travels the countryside around Roanoke, Virginia, visiting private homes of severely handicapped children and schools where the kids are mainstreamed.

Aubrey Fine places very firm limits on the young patients who come to his psychotherapy office in Pomona, California. Patients must wash their hands before they touch one of his rabbits, dogs, birds, or lizards. They must be gentle and speak in soft voices, and if the animal doesn't want to engage, they must let it go. He watches how even the rowdiest kids will not scream in the presence of the birds because, if they do, the startled birds will fly away. With the birds handling the conduct and deportment aspect of the session, real progress can be made, says Aubrey, editor of *The Handbook on Animal Assisted Therapy*, a very well thought out collection of some of the best recent research on this subject.

His warren of rooms holds his two fish tanks and a herpetarium for the lizards, a cage for the rabbit, and one for each of the four birds. "As a therapist, I'll use anything I can to get their attention," he said. "But the animals do more than that. They change my office from a threatening environment to a fascinating one." Certainly Aubrey had my attention as he was saying this. It was the only professional discussion I've ever conducted with a man who had a lizard sitting in his hair.

Aubrey treated a boy named Scott, whom he described as borderline in intelligence and suffering from a severe learning disability. He was the brunt of endless jokes by his peers and ached from the social isolation, but he really sprang to life in the presence of one of Aubrey's birds. "Birds present a wonderful metaphor in therapy," Aubrey said. "Cages, freedom, flying, beauty. The majesty of a bird is like a snowflake." The boy's family moved out of town, but they returned a few years later. When therapy resumed, Aubrey got him a bird.

Scott joined an aviary club and started to breed birds on his own. The birds gave him something to talk about, and he became more comfortable in the world. He got positive attention for his skill with them, as well as a purpose in life. What many of these troubled children lack is a sense of competence. They have failed, but they've also not had much of a chance in the first place. The best of these animal programs for children offer them a way to demonstrate their competence with animals publicly, as another way to boost their image and self-esteem.

The Green Chimneys kids dominate the local 4-H fair. In Roanoke, Mona's kids bring their animals into classrooms, too. She carefully coaches the classroom students to ask specific factual questions, which her students proudly answer. She's also encouraged the local llama breeding society to add a special needs category in their annual llama show. In coaching them for the competition, Mona is teaching them basic skill sets of motor planning, processing a sequence of movements, but they are also getting validation from a world that largely ignores them.

In the world of these troubled children, the animals connect but they also soothe and inspire, as they did in Columbine. To the Green Chimneys kids, raised on the shattered streets of the worst neighborhoods in New York City, the animals symbolize acceptance for being exactly who you are. But to Paul Kupchik, a bird-lover like Aubrey, birds further represent freedom and hope.

Green Chimneys has one of the country's largest rehabilitative centers for wounded birds of prey thanks to Paul, a first-class falconer. No tour of Green Chimneys is complete without a stroll through the aviary to the left of the main barn to view the impressive flock: Andean condor; barn, screech, and great horned owls; black and redheaded turkey vultures; ferruginous, Cooper's, kestrel, marsh, and red-tailed hawks. In giving me a personal tour, Sam Ross came to a stop in front of a favorite, a bald eagle who lost a wing in the Exxon *Valdez* oil spill. "Maybe by osmosis they will get the message that yes, handicapping conditions are bad, but if you strive hard enough, you can improve yourself," Sam said. "Wild animals don't belong in cages and kids don't belong in residential treatment facilities. But if we all work really, really hard, we can set them all free."

I visited Green Chimneys on a beautiful Saturday in June for its annual Birds of Prey Day, when people from the surrounding community are invited to the farm for a day of tours, live music, and wildlife demonstrations. The release of a rehabilitated bird is the culmination of the festivities. Paul and his helpers hoisted the bird, a red-winged hawk that had been rescued after being hit by a car on a Brooklyn expressway, up a large climbing tower in a big metal box.

Fellow falconer and Paul's friend, Robert Kennedy Jr., scaled the side of the tower and stood in the chamber at the top. He put on heavy protective gloves and gingerly opened the box, handling the bird gently, as if it were an egg. With a flourish, he opened his hands and the bird pumped his wings as they propelled him high into the sky while the crowd cheered him on. In this big public ceremony, Paul didn't shed a tear. However, when he releases a bird when one of the students moves on from Green Chimneys to the big world beyond, he does.

Paul's first rehabilitated bird lived in a very small cage Paul had built back in a time when he admits he didn't really know what he was doing. Paul had to take the bird to a veterinarian for an X ray to be assured that it was healed. But as Paul watched him flit back and forth in his little box, he wondered if when the bird was released, he'd flap his way right to the ground. The boy who was going home that day had worked with Paul to rehabilitate this bird, so as the moment approached to release him, Paul had his fingers crossed.

All the students and the staff gathered around to watch the bird go free. "I remember the kid letting the bird go and watching him take a few flaps, a few more flaps, and then start to get higher and higher and higher," Paul said. "Everybody's heart is pounding and the kid's saying, 'Come on, get up there. Go, go, go.' And then the other kids picked up on it. 'Go. Please get up. Please go. Please go. Please.' And then we realized we were on to something. For some of those kids, nothing ever meant so much."

The bird faltered for a while, stayed low, close to the trees. But at the last minute his wings started to pump with a strong, regular rhythm. He gained the altitude and was gone. Free.

Bypass Heart Problems

EACH TIME MIKE LINGENFELTER SITS in the driver's seat of his van, he touches the tiny gold angel he has pinned to the underside of the sun visor. Simultaneously with his other hand, he strokes the head of his golden retriever, Dakota, who takes the passenger seat, his front paws on the floor and his chin on the dashboard. If there is another human present, as there is this day, Dakota sits on the hump behind Mike with his head resting on the partition between the seats. Wherever he is, Mike's hand finds Dakota's head before he turns the ignition, and many times off and on during the drive. "I'm gonna be all right, Dakota," he says, threading his blunt fingers through Dakota's smooth fur. "I'm gonna be fine."

For a man who has spent his professional life as a communications engineer, placing one hand on the angel and the other on Dakota is like connecting a circuit. He believes his dog really is an angel, and you'd have to be pretty cynical to doubt him. Mike, who has severe coronary artery disease, literally cannot count the number of times Dakota has saved his life. Dakota senses when Mike is about to have a heart attack and warns him to leave stressful situations to take his medicine. "I couldn't put an emotional number or a dollar value on this dog," Mike says. "This dog is leading me through life. All I'm doing is following the dog."

This acquiescent attitude is the polar opposite to the Mike Lingenfelter at the peak of his career when he was suddenly stricken with heart disease. He'd designed the communications systems for and supervised the construction of subways in Beijing, New Delhi, Calcutta, and Riyadh, among others, in his five years at Parsons Incorporated. His bosses were so impressed with his work in 1989 that they promoted him to project engineer supervising the construction of the Red Line branch of the Los Angeles' Metro System. He and his wife Nancy, their three children launched on their own lives, had settled in Irvine, a university town forty-two miles south of Los Angeles.

The day after he'd received a clean bill of health through a flawless cardio stress test, Mike took his regular Saturday spin on his bike. He was three miles from home when he suffered a massive heart attack and fell by the side of the street. He doesn't know how long he lay on the asphalt before he regained consciousness. Using his bike as a rolling cane, he slowly made his way back. When Nancy returned from running some errands, she found her husband collapsed in the driveway. She got him in the car and raced to the nearest hospital.

The doctors at Irvine Medical Center put Mike on intravenous clot-busting drugs and attached a heart pump. They had to wait three days before he was stable enough to be transferred to Western Medical Center in Newport Beach for surgery. The angiogram they took at Western "scared the hell out of the doctors," Mike said. He had a 100 percent blockage of the left side and a 99 percent blockage on the right. They scheduled surgery for the next morning. That night, Mike suffered another heart attack. "This was the big one," he says. "This is the one when you hear them say: 'We're losing him.' " They rushed him into surgery at 4:30 A.M. for an emergency triple bypass.

When Mike left the hospital ten days after his first heart attack, he threw himself into cardio rehab, determined to be the model patient. He wanted to get right back to work. "They were always trying to get me to slow down," he remembers. No matter how slowly he walked on the treadmill, however, he suffered severe chest pains. The staff asked his cardiologist to sign a waiver so the center wouldn't be liable if he suffered a heart attack there, but his doctor refused to sign. By mutual agreement, Mike gave up rehab.

As he languished at home trying to understand the sudden turn in his fortunes, doctors told him the damage to his heart was worse than they'd first realized. In the end they decided Mike wasn't strong enough to withstand another operation. Mike resigned his job and applied for a full medical disability. Without a battle to fight or a problem to solve, he withdrew into hopelessness. "A man's role is to work and support his family," Mike said. "I had no purpose. I've been a Type A personality all my life. I've always been one hundred percent right, and that was the way it was going to be."

A Type A personality was the unspoken requirement to succeed in Mike's job. In fact, cardiologists Meyer Friedman and Ray Rosenman, who did the original research on Type A behavior and heart disease, first called it "hurry sickness." They defined Type A behavior as observable in any person who is involved in a chronic struggle to achieve more and more in less and less time.

You've either observed, lived with, or are a Type A person. The airline travelers you've seen hitting the ON button of their computer within a cat's whisker of the captain's okay sign, thumbing through a mountain of paperwork that they pull out of a pregnant briefcase, and then walking onto the jet way jawboning into a cell phone. How about soccer moms who race home from a professional job exhausted, only to find a mountain of laundry, no milk in the fridge, and three kids' afterschool activities to squeeze into approaching darkness? Even our children are becoming Type As. My daughter, Mikkel, takes a full load of honors classes in high school, is a teen leader in 4-H, takes horse riding lessons a two-and-a-half-hour drive away at least once a week, attends horse shows ten out of twelve weekends in the summer, and even takes her weekly singing lessons in a foreign country (neighboring Canada). Did I mention that she has ranch chores, sang for about a dozen community events, got her driver's license, and managed to test-drive five different boyfriends in less than a year? It's exhausting to reflect on it, let alone live it.

Mike and his peers were drawn to a life with that kind of pressure. When you ask Mike what he loved about his job, "adrenaline high" is at the top of his list. He used to leave for work every morning at 4:30 A.M. and not return until 7:30 that evening. Constructing a subway system takes four or five years, but the engineers must meet a crucial deadline every month. Mike, and the five other men at Parsons who hold his job, faced the added stress of trying to accomplish this highly sophisticated task in foreign countries where unexpected cultural differences always gummed up the works. But that was just fine with these Type As, who love to take on more responsibility than they can handle. Speeding through demanding tasks gives them a rush and they can get awfully nasty if you try to get in their way.

While productivity in our country is soaring, spirits are often sagging as our high-tech, high-intensity lifestyle takes a silent but deadly toll on our bodies. The sickness part of "hurry sickness" is that this constant state of frenzy spikes cholesterol, which lingers in the bloodstream three to four times longer in Type A people, ensuring that the lining of the arteries is continually exposed to large amounts of cholesterol. Mike and his peers prove the Type A thesis: all of them have had heart bypass operations, and so far three have suffered strokes.

Mike's wife, Nancy, was very worried as she watched her formerly vigorous, restless, and impatient husband becoming more and more withdrawn, hardly ever leaving the house. She took early retirement from her job to care for him, but her presence didn't boost his optimism or motivate him to be more active. The family doctor suggested they get a dog. He knew of a study published in 1980 that showed that heart attack sufferers who owned pets had a four times better chance of surviving one year.

This study, by James Lynch, Aaron Katcher, and Erika Friedmann, recruited ninety-six people from the University of Maryland Hospital who had recently suffered their first heart attacks, and asked if they could check in with them once a month for a year. By the end of the year, of the thirty-nine people without pets, eleven had died. Of the fifty who owned pets, only three had died. Although the petless patients represented less than half the sample, they accounted for four times more deaths. That study and those subsequently conducted to test the thesis didn't establish to a certainty how the animals helped their companions, but the researchers' guesses described the benefits of animal companionship as if they were the ultimate cardiac rehabilitation tool. Pet owners had shorter hospital stays because they wanted to get home to care for their animals. Dog owners had 8 percent fewer doctor visits, and cat owners saw the doctor 12 percent less. The pet-owning population took less medication for high blood pressure and cholesterol and didn't have as much trouble falling asleep at night.

Perhaps this was because those with dogs were significantly more active generally, scoring higher on their amount of exercise and lower in serum cholesterol, despite the fact that they tended to eat more fatty take-out food, as a 1992 Australian study of nearly six thousand cardiovascular disease sufferers found. And the beneficial effect of pets seemed to work regardless of the severity of the patient's heart disease.

In summary, a pet can be a miracle drug that keeps you healthier; home instead of hospitalized; reduces your risk of heart attacks; and keeps you healthier with a lick of a tongue, wag of a tail, or rhythmic purring. All of these benefits are available, not during doctors' hours, but around the clock. And not for a fortune, but at the price of a can of Fancy Feast or Friskies.

Patients with pets were also far more likely to stick to a cardiac rehabilitation program, according to a study conducted at the University of Texas at El Paso Psychology Department. Researchers kept tabs on seventy-nine Texas heart patients whose doctors had prescribed a rigorous twelve-week rehabilitation program: appointments four times a week for exercise, monitoring, and education. Ninety-six percent of the pet owners completed the program, compared to 77 percent of those who did not own pets. Caring for their pets gave these people a sense of responsibility and a schedule, factors useful in breaking their old bad habits, said researcher Mary M. Herrald.

Modern medicine relies on proof with a capital "P" in the form of peer-reviewed studies by top researchers in elite medical schools, looking at large populations over many years to decide if a diagnosis or treatment warrants widespread acceptance and use. If a treatment saves time, money, and lives, it becomes favored over time. For example, after studies proved that EKGs could detect heart problems and mammograms could detect cancer, doctors and patients accepted them as routine screening tools. A pet that acts as a heart attack prevention and detection machine certainly doesn't fit the traditional high standards for the medical masses, but could it be "the" answer that modern medicine, with all of its miracles, was still unable to provide Mike?

Although rehab was out of the question for Mike, the couple was cheered by the possibility that a dog might motivate him out of his slump. The couple got a golden retriever they named Abby. Abby was playful and energetic, bred to encourage Mike to get out and exercise. Her demands for attention just annoyed Mike, however. Right from the beginning, Mike thought of her as "more trouble than she was worth." He'd feed her and take her outside, but he saw it as a duty, not a joy. The doctors began medicating him for depression. "I was taking pills to get up in the morning and pills to go to bed at night. I was a vegetable," he recalled.

With Mike on disability and Nancy retired, the high cost of living in southern California was eating into their savings. In 1994, the couple moved to Texas to cut overhead and allow them to be closer to their daughter Susan and her family. They also moved to be near Southern Methodist Hospital, which has one of the best cardiac units in the country. Yet the doctor's prognosis for Mike remained poor.

As Mike languished, the creature who would change his life was languishing, too. Karen Costello, who headed up the rescue efforts for the Greater Houston Golden Retriever Club, received a call from a woman who said she'd picked up a stray golden and wanted them to take it off her hands. Karen waited at the front of the house as the owner brought out the "stray," a beautifully-cared-for dog with a dark, lustrous coat. As the two women spoke, the dog wandered into a neighbor's yard. The woman yelled sharply: "Dakota, come!" and the dog trotted obediently back.

The vet who assessed Dakota quickly established why he had been abandoned. He had a bad case of heartworms that would be expensive to treat. The vet started him on a course of heartworm medicine and Karen brought him to a foster family who would care for Dakota while Karen found him a home. Right from the start, Dakota exhibited outstanding abilities. He was eager to retrieve, a defining trait in a good service dog, and extremely sensitive to the family's emotional needs. The foster family recommended Dakota be donated to the Texas Hearing and Service Dog Association, but when vets examined Dakota, they discovered hip dysplasia, a misfit of the hip ball in the socket, which can lead to gait difficulties later in the dog's life. Texas Hearing and Service Dogs rejected Dakota and returned him to his foster family.

Just around the time of Dakota's rescue, Mike and Nancy decided to try to find another dog, one who could be trained to help Mike with menial tasks such as fetching objects for him. They asked the Golden Retriever Club if they had a suitable dog, and Karen suggested Dakota. Mike was drawn to Dakota because of his plight, which he thought of as similar to his own: rejected because of heart problems and unable to work despite his obvious aptitude.

The Friday afternoon when Mike first laid eyes on Dakota, he didn't much like what he saw: another rambunctious adolescent who'd probably prove to be as irritating as Abby, he believed. That afternoon, as Mike lay in bed, Dakota stood at the bedside nudging him with his squeaky green frog and wagging it in Mike's face. If Mike was sleeping, Dakota would nose his way underneath the covers and crawl up on his belly to again present Mike with the green frog. "This dog is such a pest," he remembers thinking. Mike and Nancy decided they'd keep him through the weekend, but agreed he was going back on Monday morning.

Mike was right. Dakota was a pest. He was watching Mike carefully, and he wasn't giving up. Saturday as Mike lay in bed, Dakota crawled underneath the sheets—this time without the frog—and lay on his side with his back up against Mike's belly. Mike reached out to hold Dakota and relaxed his body weight against him. As the two lay there, the warmth of the dog beside him calm and still for as long as Mike wanted, Dakota reached Mike some place deep inside his depression. "Dakota knows just what to do to make you comfortable," Mike says. By Sunday, Dakota was there to stay. "In the end, I decided: What the hell," Mike says. "He was my last chance."

He may, in fact, have been Mike's last chance. The cycle of depression, isolation, and inactivity that had Mike in its grip leads to even less activity, thereby further damaging the heart. A recent study of 350 heart patients by doctors at Duke University Medical Center demonstrated that the higher the patients scored on a depression scale, the lower was the reactivity of their hearts. Among the clinically depressed heart patients—such as Mike before Dakota—one in four rated themselves as extremely inactive, as compared with one in fourteen for those who weren't depressed. Depressed people averaged only half as much time engaged in moderate activity such as walking.

Isolation leads to depression, and depression leads to elevated stress hormones, which lowers heart resiliency, according to a study by Dr. Robert Carney of Washington University Medical School in St. Louis.

Another study, by the Montreal Heart Institute, found that depression raises the odds of dying from a second heart attack, particularly if the individual walks less than a block a day. Others are taking note. Knowing that pets motivate people to exercise, fight depression, reduce blood pressure, and help prevent heart disease, the Midland Life Insurance Company of Columbus, Ohio, even gives a premium discount to pet owners.

One thing a pet can do is get you to walk that block a day and maybe more, which is precisely what Dakota did for Mike. His reaction to Dakota was a 180-degree difference to that he'd had to Abby. While Abby, who now was Nancy's dog, had harassed and cajoled Mike into finally taking her out, Mike was happy to take Dakota for a walk. "Abby has love like all goldens, but Dakota has compassion. I never thought you could have this kind of closeness," Mike said.

Dakota's dignity and his responsiveness to obedience training impressed Mike. Within a few months, Mike and Dakota had enrolled in an obedience program at the Second Baptist Church. They set out to get him certified as a service dog by the Delta Society, and got him a Canine Good Citizenship Award through the local American Kennel Club. This increasing activity had a salubrious effect on Mike. Six months after he got Dakota, Mike was off all the tranquilizers and antidepressants he'd been taking for three years. Mike was still experiencing severe chest pains four to six times a month, and occasionally three or four in a day. These incidents were far less frequent than when he'd been home alone, however.

As soon as Dakota got his service dog vest, the pair began speaking at schools. Mike used himself and Dakota as an example of the incredible effect service dogs could have on the life of someone who was gravely ill. That fall, they addressed an elementary school. Mike was well into his spiel on the excellent behavior and steadfast obedience of service dogs when Dakota started acting up. Although Dakota was trained to sit quietly on the floor at his feet as Mike spoke, Dakota laid his head on Mike's lap and stared steadily at him.

Mike was embarrassed that Dakota would not follow his command to sit and stay, but he wanted to finish his presentation. As he continued, Dakota got more insistent. He started poking Mike with his nose. Finally Mike couldn't take it anymore and cut his lecture short. He and Dakota were in the corridor heading toward the parking lot when Mike was felled by a heart attack. When he came to, the first thing he felt was Dakota licking his face. "He smelled that heart attack. He had tried to warn me," Mike says. "He was licking that smell off."

Mike's cardiologist, Dr. Eugene Henderson, supposes, as do others familiar with the acute senses of dogs, that Dakota does smell a heart attack coming on. When the heart muscle is damaged, enzymes build up in the bloodstream five to eight hours before the attack. After an attack, doctors test your blood for the presence of these chemicals to confirm that you've had one. Although some have supposed that Dakota notices a change in Mike's behavior, Mike disagrees. On several occasions, Dakota has come in from another room to alert Mike that he's in trouble and give him time to take his medicine before the heart attack takes hold. As Mike's cardiologist describes Dakota's life-saving role, he's a fire dog: "It's a lot easier to put the fire out when it's just a match instead of when the whole house is on fire."

Whatever Dakota is sensing, the certainty that another creature was so attuned to the changes in his body, so alert to him getting himself into danger, allowed Mike to regain the life he had missed so much while he was ill. He returned to work at Parsons, designing communications systems for subways in Pittsburgh and Buffalo. He began to travel again, and he brought Dakota with him wherever he went.

One day during a meeting on a troubled project, colleague Rob Knoebber saw Dakota at work.

"The project was at a rough place and no one wanted to take the blame," Knoebber recalls. "Voices were raised. Ultimatums were laid down and Mike was right in the middle of it. Dakota came up to Mike and bumped him. He let Mike know it wasn't a safe place."

After Dakota led Mike out of the room, the tone of the meeting changed. "We took a look at the way we were behaving and all got a grip on ourselves," Knoebber said. "Dakota kind of pulled the plug on the whole thing."

In that action, Dakota performed a more generalized version of the same protection he offered to Mike. As disagreements build to arguments and tensions rise, the body senses danger. The reaction to stress is basic, animalistic, and instinctual—a snap assessment of which course of action offers the best odds for survival, called the fight-or-flight response. To get the body ready to fight or flee, breathing accelerates as adrenaline pumps through the bloodstream. The muscles tighten and blood pressure spikes as the heart accelerates—jumping ten to thirty beats per minute in the space of a single heartbeat—to pump blood from the gut to the muscles.

This powerful hormonal response was an advantage for our primitive ancestors who could be jumped by a man-eating saber-toothed tiger hiding behind an adjacent rock. But life in the age of technology has turned it into a health liability, when the danger we face is being jumped by a quota-seeking sales associate in a pinstriped suit. With twenty-first century threats *de jour*, our bodies jump into hyperalert in response to situations where fighting or fleeing isn't the reasonable reaction. As Harvard cardiologist Dr. Herbert Benson notes in his book *The Relaxation Response*, the fight-or-flight reaction is increasingly brought on by events that merely call for a change in attitude. It's what the late naturalist Paul Shepard characterized as "turning the predator mind on the non-prey world."

Today we're all trying to do more and more in less and less time. Talking on the phone and driving the car is commonplace, as is talking on the phone and driving while bolting down a fast-food meal and skipping CD tracks with a greasy finger. It's celebrated as multitasking, and is considered vital to increased productivity, profitability, and economic survival.

And forget about being idle for a few hours. Most of us get anxious if we're idle for more than a few seconds. I live in the wilderness, yet from anywhere in the house I can hear the fax tone singing over the sound of the birds and the cheery robotic voice announcing "You've got mail" on one of my four computers. The sounds of technology don't evoke the same childhood anticipation as when the mailman pulled up to our rural mailbox and the whole family raced to see who was trying to communicate with our family. I could characterize the modern lifestyle as the microwave minute: the minute that takes too long.

It used to be when I warmed my coffee in the microwave, I pressed the timer for one minute. While the seconds ticked by, maddeningly slowly, I paced the floor fretting about what I should be doing. If I could stop fixating on the clock and turn my head forty-five degrees, I'd be looking at the tall, conifer-covered mountains that rim the valley below our deck. There's usually a breeze coming south through the valley toward our house. Every day, if you bother to look, you'll see eagles and hawks making breathtaking swoops to the valley floor. But my mind was so packed with thoughts, I didn't look. Fifteen or so seconds before that minute was up, the coffee was warm enough, I'd figure, and I'd grab it and head back to work.

A perfect example of the fight-or-flight response readying one to act when no action is possible is "fighting traffic." Wedged in side by side with other frustrated drivers in a freeway traffic jam, your body feels ready for a fight. It certainly is a stressful situation, but it's a situation you can't do anything about. You inch forward slowly, quick to rage if anyone cuts in front of you. Your body is all revved up with no place to blow.

Cell phones alone could be responsible for the proportion of workers who described themselves as "feeling highly stressed," which the American Institute on Stress estimates has more than doubled since 1985—the year cell phones hit the market—to 1995. Cell phones, pagers, and laptops have essentially obliterated the barrier between public and private space, giving us no respite from our own work, and increasing encroachment on the work and private lives of others. Ever had a meal with someone who was trying to be polite by not answering his or her cell phone? They twitch like addicts going through withdrawal.

For example, you're standing in the supermarket considering the five rows of shelf space devoted to salad dressing, when another customer comes up beside you talking on the cell phone. She's having an intimate, detailed discussion of her mother's health with some medical professional. "What's the white cell count? Do you think it's leukemia?" Simultaneously your heart extends sympathy and the desire to connect, while your mind wishes you didn't have to hear this deeply personal dilemma. You don't know whether to offer her a handkerchief or ask her to leave. So you do nothing. You stand there unable to move or to figure out what to buy.

This is a circumstance that fits cardiologists A. M. Ostfeld and R. B. Shekelle's description of the stress-addled modern life, in which increasingly you are in situations where you really don't know how to react. The fact that appropriate behavior isn't "prescribed and validated by tradition" raises your stress level in a heartbeat. When the body goes into alert too often, it's a murderous circumstance for people with bad hearts, and it leads to heart attacks and strokes. The more often stressful situations confront you, the quicker your body leaps into overdrive.

Cardiovascular disease kills half of all Americans, men and women.

Medically speaking, Nancy should be just as concerned about herself as Mike, as each year more than eleven times as many women die of cardiovascular disease than breast cancer. Nearly a million of us each year die of heart disease and another 600,000 suffer a stroke, a third of whom die within a few months. Heart disease is also the leading cause of premature death as more than a third of heart attacks occur in those under the age of sixty-five. Heart attacks are twice as deadly in women than men. In 1999, the American Heart Association estimated that another fifty-nine million Americans—one in five—lived with some form of cardiovascular disease, with fifty million of them suffering from high blood pressure.

Recent guidelines published in the *Journal of the American Medical Association* say that the twelve million Americans who take cholesterol-lowering drugs such as Lipitor, Zocor, and Mevacor could eventually increase to thirty-six million, or one in five Americans. This would increase those people's prescription costs to $100 per month—perhaps far cheaper than the $105 billion it costs to treat heart disease. Drug companies and research institutes spend billions trying to find a medication that will lower cholesterol and blood pressure by even twenty points, exactly what pets do for practically nothing.

What a dog like Dakota offers is a basic tool in stress reduction: a focus on something outside yourself. Anxiety decreases your ability to attend to the world around you; you get bound up in your own head. Studies have shown that this calming effect is not limited to dogs. A study conducted by Aaron Katcher and Alan Beck at the University of Pennsylvania dental school placed patients scheduled for tooth extraction in a waiting room with a fish tank or a poster of a mountain scene. Those who contemplated the fish tank exhibited less anxiety during surgery and had a better subjective memory of it than those who viewed the mountain scene. Katcher and Beck suggested that watching the fish move about the tank created a modified form of meditation, but they also speculated a more intriguing secondary reason for the patients' reduced level of stress.

The sight of undisturbed animals and plants is a symbol of peace and harmony buried deep in our evolutionary history and supported in popular culture, they wrote. The aquarium, with its swaying plants and calm fish, is a contained but reassuring image of the Peaceable Kingdom that brings us instantly into a meditative state.

Living with a pet full-time has an even greater effect on stress reduction in a population whose general level of stress is extremely high. Dr. Karen Allen, a medical researcher at the State University of New York at Buffalo, studied the effect of pet ownership on the most anxious population she could identify: forty-eight New York City stockbrokers.

All of the subjects in this study made more than $200,000 a year, lived alone, and suffered from high blood pressure. A blood pressure reading of less than 140/110 is considered normal, but these subjects' blood pressure averaged 165/110 at rest. In the first session with the subjects, Allen and her colleagues asked them to complete two stressful tasks: counting backwards from seventeen, and giving a five-minute speech trying to talk their way out of a shoplifting charge. Their blood pressure jumped on average 182/126 after completing the math task, and to 184/126 at the end of the speech. When the subjects were given an ACE inhibitor, a common blood pressure reduction medicine, their pressure dropped back into the normal range with scores averaging 122/76.

The researchers then randomly instructed half of the stockbrokers to get a dog or cat. Six months later they were asked to complete another stressful test. Allen had them improvise a five-minute discussion with a client who was furious because the stockbroker had just lost $86,000 of the client's money. Those with pets experienced only half the blood pressure increase of those without.

The blood pressure scores for these highly stressed stockbrokers demonstrated that even when separated from their pets for hours, overall their cardiovascular system was still receiving the beneficial effect of the contact. After all, in addition to the visual cue that all is right with the world when they see their cat sleeping on his favorite part of the windowsill, having a pet offers tactile encouragement to relax.

In *The Relaxation Response*, Dr. Herbert Benson offered a home recipe for stress reduction: get in a comfortable position in a quiet place. Clear thoughts from your head by finding something outside yourself on which to focus. This simple blood pressure-reducing formula, similar to meditation, is naturally available while petting your animal. The health benefits of petting are even greater, however. Instead of focusing on a spot on the wall or repeating the same word over and over to dull the mind of thought, with a pet you receive the well-established health benefits of contact, a phenomenon which is called, oddly enough, "the effect of person."

More than forty years ago, Dr. W. Horsley Gantt, a researcher at Johns Hopkins University, coined that phrase to describe the powerful effect that human contact has on the cardiovascular response of animals. Gantt was the only American disciple of the Russian scientist Ivan Petrovich Pavlov, the man who tested conditioned response on dogs by isolating them in a chamber, ringing a bell, and then feeding them. After a time, Pavlov's dogs would start to salivate upon hearing the bell.

Researchers in Gantt's laboratory were testing for a more positive conditioned response. They isolated dogs in small chambers and regularly monitored their blood pressure. When a person first entered the chamber, the dog's blood pressure rose quickly. But as the person petted the dog, the animals' blood pressure and heart rate dropped by as much as 50 percent. Nonthreatening contact, even from someone the dogs didn't know, quickly calmed them down.

In the early sixties, Gantt extended the research to see if the effect on the animals was as strong in a stressful situation. In this experiment, the dogs received an electrical shock to their forelimb without warning and technicians recorded their heart rate increase. After establishing the dogs' average response, the shock was administered while the dogs were being petted. While some expected the human would get bitten, the opposite turned out to be true. The contact with another creature appeared to lessen the perception of the pain. The dog's heart rate increased only half as much while being petted.

This isn't so surprising, if you think about it in human-to-human terms. A mother rushes to her child who is sobbing and distraught because she has just tumbled off her bicycle and scraped a knee. The mother gathers her daughter up in her arms and presses her against her chest, enveloping her as she rocks back and forth, cooing reassurance. The child relaxes against her, absorbs her mother's warmth and strength, and suddenly it doesn't seem to hurt so much.

One of the young researchers in Gannt's lab was James Lynch, who with Katcher and Friedmann later conducted that groundbreaking study of how pets increase your chances of surviving after a heart attack. Lynch spent the rest of his career studying how loneliness is a huge contributing factor to heart disease, a case he makes most persuasively in his book, *A Cry Unheard*.

Working at Johns Hopkins and as a member of the faculty of the University of Maryland Medical School, Lynch studied the population of heart attack patients. Many of them were lonely men and women who could lie for days and even weeks without a visitor, their families scattered all over the country, their lives devoid of contact, let alone companionship. The healing power of touch on these people was evident even through the briefest contact. Lynch found that the touch of a nurse taking a patient's pulse could temporarily settle a dangerous arrhythmia.

While working on the 1980 study of pet ownership and heart patients, Lynch found more proof of the debilitating lifestyle of these cardiac patients. Some of the patients they surveyed had their heart attacks within six months of losing a spouse. Many others were confirmed loners. One woman said she didn't know the name of anyone in the neighborhood she'd lived in for forty-five years, and one man noted that he did not recognize a single person on his block. Animal companionship proved to be more than just a way to chase the blues away for people like these; it was a lifesaver. Those with pets, the Australian study discovered, naturally had a better social life. Nearly 60 percent of them made friends through their pets, and 62 percent said their pets made conversation with a visitor easier.

The researcher who worked with Katcher and Lynch on the study was Erika Friedmann, now a professor at the Department of Health and Nutrition Sciences at Brooklyn College. In 1995 she decided to conduct the study again with a larger sample of people and more refined measurement techniques.

She recruited 392 patients who had suffered heart attacks and were participating in the Cardiac Arrhythmia Suppression Trial and tested them with a sophisticated battery of psychological assessment tests to establish their social support and mental health. One year later, the results for this larger population were even more dramatic than the 1980 study. Of the eighty-seven people who owned a dog, only one had died. Of the 282 who didn't own dogs, nineteen had, making those who owned a dog *eight times* more likely to survive one year after a heart attack. The top four factors for one-year's survival were the strength of the heart, absence of diabetes, regularity of heartbeat, and owning a dog. Ownership of a dog was the number one psychosocial factor in survival.

Arlene Williams, a veterinary hospital manager and former human ICU nurse, knows the power of animal contact. She worked for nine years with cardiologist Dr. Peter Thom in Arroyo Grande, California, where they routinely wrote prescriptions for people to get a dog, cat, or bird. Arlene had noticed that many of their cardiology patients were coming in once a week, even though they only needed to come in once every six months. She surmised that many of the "little old ladies" were lonely and needed companionship. Knowing the problem and the treatment, Arlene began to suggest that these patients get a pet. Their answer, of course, was "My landlord, my neighbors, family, spouse, whatever, would never permit me to do that." That prompted Arlene to ask: "What if Dr. Thom wrote you a prescription, for a specific type of pet, a very specific pet prescription?" To that they responded, "Why, that would probably make all of the difference in the world!"

Now all Arlene had to do was convince her nonpet-loving boss to write the prescriptions. Arlene would sit with the patients and determine what species and breed of pet would be best and, once they agreed, would get an initially skeptical Dr. Thom to write the prescription. She told the patients, "If anyone gives you problems about honoring the prescription at any time, call me and I'll personally see to it that the doctor explains his rationale for prescribing the pet." No one ever called to dispute the prescription, and in fact, several patients got refills in the form of other pets. Arlene says, "Dr. Thom was amazed at how powerfully pets helped our patients."

Connecticut cardiologist Dr. Stephen Sinatra, author of *Heartbreak and Heart Disease*, has found this to be true in his patient population. As a result, he prescribes pets just like he prescribes medications for about 15 percent of his patients, because he's seen how effective they can be to connect to the lonely and motivate a new routine. "When patients have lost a spouse or live alone, a lot of them can't make a vital connection in their lives," Dr. Sinatra said. "You'd be surprised how many people can connect to a pet. If they pour a lot of loving energy into a pet, the pet pours it back."

The chief advantage of animals as agents of calm, Lynch believes, is that they do not talk. His research indicates that the act of speaking increases blood pressure dramatically, depending on who the audience is and how the speaker is talking. Those speaking quickly and breathlessly experience elevated blood pressure, as do those who are talking to someone they perceive to be of higher social status. Medication, by and large, does not block the elevation of blood pressure that comes from talking. The only thing that can help is focusing on something outside yourself. "Those things that get us outside ourselves immediately elicit the calming of the body," Lynch said.

For that very reason, Dr. Sinatra started bringing his dogs to the office more than a decade ago. He has three: a Norwegian elkhound named Charlie whom he calls a "love machine," and two chows, Chewie (short for Chewbacca) and Kooa. The presence of a dog in the room makes the doctor-patient dialogue better, he believes. "Sometimes you get people who drain your energy," he says. "You can feel as though you are being sucked dry. I pet the dog. The patient pets the dog and begins to tell his story. When I'm petting the dog, it opens my heart. And when my heart is open, I'm a much more effective healer."

In the anxious and sterile world of the doctor's office, the best focal points come from the natural world, even if the human has nothing more to look at than fish swimming in a tank. If you are lucky enough to be a patient of Dr. Sinatra's, you get a soothing touch that offers understanding at a primitive level. When you are using words to explain your body to another, the effort can elicit the fear that you will not be understood, Lynch says. Animals never judge and are predictable and accepting, the opposite of fight or flight. Their relaxed, fearless, and constant presence says "stay and play." Or as Mike Lingenfelter says: "If you talk to people, you get all the wrong answers. When you talk to Dakota, you get nothing but right answers."

As time wore on, Dakota was certainly satisfying Mike's need for contact with his constant presence and his attentiveness to the world around Mike. He alerted three of Mike's coworkers, one of whom had a heart attack a few hours after Dakota warned him. The other two were later determined to have heart disease. After a time, Dakota began sleeping right in the center of the bed between Mike and Nancy. Nancy doesn't complain because Dakota has demonstrated that he can save her husband's life, even if she can't.

In July 1999 around five in the morning, Dakota woke up suddenly. He sensed something wasn't right with Mike and tried to wake him. Mike didn't stir, even though Dakota tugged at his sleeve and nudged him repeatedly. When Dakota couldn't get Mike to respond, he woke Nancy. She rolled over in bed and tried to wake her husband but he didn't rouse. Frantically, she called 911. When the paramedics arrived a few minutes later and checked Mike's blood pressure, they found it hovering at 60/38. With those low numbers, as Dr. Henderson puts it, if it hadn't been for Dakota, "Mike wouldn't have said hello to his wife that morning."

Dakota's ability to warn of Mike's heart attacks is a rare gift. There are other dogs who perform this service for their companions, but their numbers are not huge. Dakota's real gift to Mike started long before that day in the elementary school. As with other animals who help bring their companions back to health after a heart attack, Dakota first gave Mike friendship. His simple, nonjudgmental companionship soothed Mike's stress and brought him out of his isolation. Then Dakota got Mike to move again, bringing him out into the world where he showed Mike he still had a role, a mission, and a purpose.

Although we can try to quantify this Bond with studies and statistics, it all comes back to the relationship with an animal reminding the human there is a reason to go on living. As James Lynch writes of this cross-species bond in *A Cry Unheard*: "There is a will to live and that will is fueled by human concern, by human and animal companionship, and by our relationship to the rest of the natural living world."

And nowhere was the depth of this cross-species Bond more dramatically demonstrated than when Mike Lingenfelter discovered that Dakota had cancer.

Cancer Cures—How Pets Are Giving People a Second Chance

SOMETHING ABOUT THE BOND BETWEEN Mike Lingenfelter and Dakota embodied everything that the relationship between a human and an animal could be. Mike had rescued Dakota from a life of neglect and Dakota, in turn, had brought Mike back to life with his ability to warn Mike he was about to have a heart attack. Once Mike was up and about in the world again, he wanted to show others how pivotal a strong, loving relationship with an animal can be for human health. Human-animal Bond organizations and the national media recognized it instantly. In 1999, Dakota was named the Assistance Dog of the Year by the Delta Society, got a place in the Texas Animal Hall of Fame, and by 2000, he'd been featured on Animal Planet. Patty Neger, a producer for *Good Morning America*, where I appear as a veterinary contributor, spotted Mike and Dakota in an article in *Men's Health* magazine and arranged to feature them. She was about to send a crew to Texas to film them when she got a call from a very shaken-up Mike, saying that maybe the film crew shouldn't come. Dakota had lymphatic cancer.

A week earlier, Mike had noticed that Dakota was moping around, drinking tremendous amounts of water, and not eating very well. His veterinarian, Dr. Harold Krug, diagnosed lymphoma and prescribed chemotherapy, but he advised Mike that his best friend and savior had only up to six months to live. Mike was devastated. He and Nancy had stayed up all night crying at the thought of losing Dakota. Patty called me in tears to ask if I knew anyone who could help.

"Is he willing to travel?" I asked.

"I think Mike would do anything to save this dog," Patty said.

"Then tell him he's got to get Dakota to Ft. Collins, Colorado," I said.

Of all twenty-seven veterinary schools in the United States where I've lectured on the Bond, the place I most enjoy is Colorado State University (CSU) College of Veterinary Medicine in Ft. Collins, Colorado. The drive from Denver to Ft. Collins—running parallel to the Rocky Mountains along the eastern front—feels like a journey to veterinary medicine's Mt. Everest. Although I am an affiliate faculty member at the vet school, my closest ties are to the college's Animal Cancer Center (ACC), one of the country's premier research institutes for human and animal cancer.

Cancer is the second leading cause of death for humans, but it hits animals even harder. Half of dogs and a third of cats will die of cancer, compared to a quarter of humans. Although animal cancer varies in incidence and frequency from human cancer, the way the cancer responds to chemotherapy and radiation is identical, says Dr. Stephen J. Withrow, the center's chief of clinical oncology. Steve has trained at the Mayo Clinic, and is the only veterinarian admitted among the doctors in the Muscular-Skeletal Tumor Society, a prestigious research association. In the past twenty years, the National Institutes of Health has provided $30 million in research grants to ACC, an institution that has conducted crucial research on innovations in bone cancer, chemotherapy delivery systems, and the use of heat and radiation.

The doctors at the center see 1,500 new patients a year, and these form the basis of their research. The center is known for fast-track treatment of its patients. The standard of care for humans doesn't permit the aggressive treatments the veterinarians at the center can employ. In the delicate balancing act of treating cancer with chemotherapy and radiation—how to give enough to kill the cancer, but not so much that you harm the patient—the animals are truly laying down their lives for us.

The veterinarians stay up to date on the latest research in human cancer, and mindfully tinker with their animal patients' dosages of radiation and chemotherapy, immune system care, and nutrition to try to establish which combinations offer the most hope for all. And most important, the research is not performed on animals raised to be killed for experiments. They don't inflict cancer on an animal and then include him or her in a clinical trial. They take our critically ill companions, animals that other vets may have given up for gone, and try to give both humans and pets another chance. For this reason, they deal not just with the clinical side of the disease, but the emotional.

"Cancer is a disease of emotion," says Dr. Greg Ogilvie, director of the center's oncology research lab. "It's a disease of shadows and hallways—the shadows of all the people you've known who died of it, your relatives and friends. Cancer represents the summit of the lack of hope."

Part of the healing power of pets is their capacity to make the atmosphere safe for emotions, the spiritual side of healing. Whatever you're feeling, you can express it around your pet. Let it out, let it go, and not be judged for it. In that way, we don't have to censor ourselves around our beloved four-legged friends, nor do we censor our feelings for them when they get sick. Beyond the medical advances taking place at ACC, what has always impressed me is the staff's capacity to face the emotional impact of disease, something that all too frequently is shoved under the rug in the treatment of cancer in humans. "When you know your caregiver is afraid and is being touched by that fear, it hurts both. We care for the pet parent as well as the patient," Greg said.

While many other veterinary schools have magnificent new brick and concrete edifices, CSU looks more like a well-lived-in home crammed with too many family members. The waiting room of ACC is a bustling place with a pleasant, upbeat atmosphere, despite the severity of the disease that brings everyone together. After all, people are with their animals. They have a mechanism for connection, a peer group that understands their dilemma, and the relief that they are doing everything they can to save their friend. It's not uncommon for people to drive all night from some place very far away to bring their pet to ACC. The day of my recent visit, the long-distance champ was a man from Vancouver who'd gone two and a half days without sleep to drive his dog to the center. The other thing ACC offers is hope. The people who bring their pets to ACC know the doctors are using the very latest and the most aggressive treatments possible.

The first thing Greg noticed about Dakota was the grayness around him. "Cancer causes changes in the body that sap the energy, the strength," Greg said. The other thing he spotted instantly was Dakota's little green frog, the same talisman that he'd used years earlier to nudge Mike out of bed and encourage him to live again. "Dakota never left Mike's side, but he greeted me with his frog in his mouth," Greg recalls. "He was sick and low, but still he was saying, 'Let's engage.'"

Dakota's tumor filled up a third of his chest and had spread to the thymus and the lymph nodes, suppressing his immune system. The problem with treating lymphoma is its location in the chest cavity. In delivering the amount of radiation and chemotherapy needed to arrest the cancer, the doctor risks damaging the heart and the lungs. "You want to focus the radiation therapy on the chest to get that cancer under control as fast as possible before it develops resistance," Greg said. "It was a balance between providing focused treatment, compassion, and preserving his ability to still help Mike."

Dakota underwent small doses of radiation ten to fifteen minutes a day Monday through Friday and weekly doses of chemotherapy. Greg also prescribed drugs to protect Dakota's heart and lungs and nutrients to expand and strengthen the immune system. Meanwhile Mike was getting a lot of pressure from his employer to go back to work. The company was sympathetic for a while, but wouldn't permit Mike to stay in Ft. Collins for the six weeks it took to treat Dakota. When Mike went back to Texas to work, Greg took Dakota into his home. "At first he'd come home and flop down," Greg recalls. Then the treatment took hold and he began to flourish. "Dakota did extremely well in therapy," Greg observed. "He just places his heart, his being, and his physical presence in your hands."

While Dakota was flourishing, Mike wasn't doing so well without him. Despite the fact that Greg called Mike a couple times a day, Mike needed Dakota at his side. His cardiologist, Dr. Eugene Henderson, was really worried. "When Dakota was gone in Colorado, Mike's health deteriorated," Dr. Henderson says. "He didn't get out as much and gained weight."

When the treatment was complete and Greg couldn't find any more signs of cancer in Dakota, Greg and his family invited Mike over for dinner and reluctantly gave Dakota back. "Even the darn guinea pig loved Dakota," Greg said, noting that some of Dakota's toys are still stashed around the Ogilvie home waiting for Dakota to visit. Although

Greg doesn't like to use the "C" word, as in "cured," eighteen months later Dakota remains in remission. Mike recently retired and he and his family have moved to Alabama, where he works occasionally as a consultant for his former employer. When he does work, Dakota always comes along.

Although Greg says every one of his patients is special to him, there are only a few that demonstrate the Bond as dramatically as Mike and Dakota. "Dakota is Mike's angel, and vice versa," Greg says. "There is a watchfulness and a kinship and a benevolence that cannot be described." The other example Greg cites of the Bond manifesting itself at its best through cancer is Bill Johnson and his dog, Max. Bill's tenacity and generosity have resulted in what potentially can help ACC take a big stride forward in cancer research for both species.

Bill Johnson's specialty in business was turning ailing companies around. By the time he retired in 1992, he wanted to step away from the rat race. He resigned the chairmanship of a Fortune 500 company and moved to Colorado and got Max, a golden retriever like Dakota. He and Max took to the mountains hiking, cross-country skiing, and rock climbing, with the unexpected side benefit of a miraculous spiritual transformation in this hard-bitten businessman.

As the stress drained out of his body, other mainstays of Bill's world started to crumble. His marriage ended and Bill was diagnosed with colon cancer, which fortunately was caught at a very early stage. Still, Bill had to have part of his colon removed and underwent chemotherapy with the unflagging companionship of Max. "Max was my Buddha, my teacher, and my healer," he says. "It wasn't just his love that was healing but the acceptance and the positive attitude toward life. There was not a negative bone in his body."

Six months after Bill's cancer treatment, Max started to tire easily. He wanted to lie down while they were cross-country skiing, and he started getting a little short of breath. But, as he was only five years old, Bill never suspected Max had cancer. When the vet diagnosed a sizeable lymphoma in his chest, Bill flew Max immediately to ACC and Dr. Greg Ogilvie. He felt terrible, as if in some way he'd let Max down. He told Greg he didn't care how inconvenient it was or how much it cost, he wanted to try *everything* to save him. Greg used a combination of natural therapies and radiation similar in spirit but different in specifics to how he'd successfully treated Dakota. After two months of treatment, the second member of the Johnson family beat back cancer.

For Bill as well as for Max, their doctors knew the cancer hadn't come back, but no test could pronounce them cured. The fight against cancer became a team effort for them. They were codependent in the best sense, united to live a lifestyle that offered both the best chance for survival. Bill had read thirty books about alternative healing methods for cancer and developed a very strict diet, which he modified for Max. He put Max on some of the same herbs and supplements he'd been using, and went so far as to consult with natural healing guru Dr. Andrew Weil for advice on Max's diet. Bill was keenly interested in anything new in early detection and pinpointing the precise location of cancer. Bill asked Greg if he knew of any researchers working in this area, and Greg suggested Dr. Doug Collins, radiologist at the Mayo Clinic, who was experimenting with vitamin B12 as a cancer-seeking missile.

A cancer cell sucks up B12 preferentially. The more aggressive the tumor is, the faster it absorbs B12. When tagged with a radioactive isotope, Doug used B12 to pinpoint the location of a tumor and assess its tenacity by imaging it with a sophisticated nuclear camera.

Traditionally, the effectiveness of cancer treatment is assessed by changes in anatomy—i.e., is the lump getting bigger or smaller? Doug Collins used B12 to track its biochemical processes; how fast the cancer was metabolizing the B12. If the tumor was metabolizing B12 hungrily, the images would show up bright white, reflecting the heat of the biochemical process. Once he got a bead on the cancer, Doug attached a different radioactive isotope to the B12, one designed to kill the cancer. With the vitamin as a delivery system, the radiation would go directly to where it was needed. The nuclear images showed immediately if the treatment was taking hold. The B12 delivery mechanism was like shooting a laser beam at point-blank range where you can't miss versus using a shotgun to shoot at a target through a dense fog.

Greg was so intrigued by Doug's work, he contacted him to offer the patients at ACC as research subjects. Doug, in turn, was very excited about working with Greg and having a chance to use the treatment on naturally developing cancers in real patients instead of cancer induced in a mouse thigh. He also loved the atmosphere. "The professional attitude, the excitement the workers have, and the dedication has a similar feel to what we have at Mayo," Doug said. "It felt like home."

They imaged a few animals on ACC's 1975 nuclear camera which, despite its primitive technology, detected the B12 lighting up the cancer. For the purposes of his research, Doug needed ACC to have a camera that cost $700,000. When Bill Johnson heard about this, he organized a meeting with administrators from CSU, Doug, and Greg to brainstorm about a way to raise the money for a new camera for the center. The timetable for acquiring the camera sped up dramatically when, a month after this meeting, Max got sick again.

Bill brought Max in for a checkup and the vet in Tucson discovered a tumor the size of a golf ball in the right atrium of Max's heart, a cancer unrelated to his lymphoma. The vet gave Max only a few days to live. Bill brought Max back to ACC that afternoon, where they decided against open-heart surgery because the operation would most likely kill him. The tumor was creating tremendous pressure on his heart. Max wasn't getting enough blood flow and plasma was backing up in his chest cavity. Greg gave him doses of thalidomide to slow the tumor and chemotherapy. Max's love for Bill was the only thing that was keeping him alive, Greg said.

Bill rented a suite at a nearby hotel and, though he had a nice bedroom, slept on a mattress on the floor next to Max so he could monitor his breathing. He bought a child's bright red wagon with removable sides in which Max rode down the elevator to the car. Meanwhile Bill was desperately trying to find a way to get two bureaucracies—CSU and the Mayo Clinic—to move fast enough to save Max.

Max was admitted to CSU on February 6, and by March 6 Bill Johnson had worked out a deal to take one of the Mayo Clinic's old cameras and transfer it to CSU while they acquired a more modern model to replace it. Bill put up $400,000 of the money for the Mayo Clinic; another research institute affiliated with Mayo contributed $165,000, and ACC pledged to raise the rest of the money.

It took Bill almost a month to put the deal together, excruciatingly slow for him but lightning-quick for Mayo and CSU. Normally it takes three weeks to get one of these cameras installed. The institutions agreed to the deal on Wednesday afternoon, and by Friday the camera was on its way to CSU. Bill got the cell phone number of the truck driver and convinced him to drive through the night. He persuaded the installation crew to be standing by when the camera arrived at 3:00 A.M. Saturday. The camera was up and running by Monday evening—normally installation takes ten days—and by Tuesday Doug Collins had flown down from Minnesota to examine nuclear images of Max's tumor.

Doug didn't like what he was seeing. The tumor filled up 80 percent of Max's right ventricle. Greg was applying to the state for special permission to do experimentally aggressive chemotherapy when it seemed like Max was starting to give up.

One day on the way back to the hotel, Bill looked at Max in the backseat and saw how sad and tired he was. Still, Bill wanted to try to get him through one more treatment. "To turn around businesses, you have to be able to convince people to do the impossible," Bill said. "I was so focused on not giving up." Bill's friend went to the back of the car to get Max when they arrived at the hotel and saw that he wasn't breathing. They rushed Max to ACC, where emergency room veterinarians used heart paddles to try to revive Max, but he was gone. At the autopsy, Greg saw that Max's tumor filled the whole chamber of his heart.

When I tell the story of how hard Bill worked and how much money he spent to try to give Max more years, people think Bill is crazy. After all, Max was just a dog. But Bill is unashamed and unconflicted. "What would you do for your best friend?" he asked. "Someone who is true to you and wonderful to you, and you have been accepted as his world, totally a hundred percent. He does it with the belief that you're going to take care of him, too. If you really feel that heart connection, it says to you that you must do everything you can. Other people can't afford the money. But I could, so why not?"

Bill is proud of Max's legacy because, as with many things in animal cancer, a few years down the line what ACC is doing with this camera will have an impact on human cancer. In fact, research on animals that took place at ACC in the late 1980s has moved forward to be used in cutting-edge treatments for humans today, as the story of a dog from one small town in Colorado demonstrates.

Chieko, a big, bounding cross between a St. Bernard and a German shepherd, started out in life weighing fifteen pounds. By the time she was fully grown, she stood six feet tall on her hind legs and weighed 123 pounds. She was a gentle giant, known to every kid in the Herrick family's neighborhood in Wheat Ridge, Colorado, for her incredible spirit of play. She was up for hiking any hour of the day, and loved backpacking trips and cross-country skiing. If you couldn't find her, chances were if you just followed the sound of children's laughter in the street, you'd find Chieko right in the middle of it. Connie Herrick remembers trying to find Chieko to comfort her the winter afternoon after she'd been spayed. She searched all over the house and finally found her outside romping with some kids. "No woman right after a hysterectomy would be out playing in the snow," Connie said.

When she came home from Christmas shopping in December 1988, Chieko greeted Connie sedately. She limped toward Connie and, after a brief wiggle and kiss, collapsed at the bottom of the stairs. Connie noticed a big bump on Chieko's left leg and she and her husband Rohn rushed Chieko in to the veterinarian, who diagnosed osteosarcoma, an aggressive bone cancer that typically develops in the larger breeds of dogs and taller humans. The vet offered two choices. They could amputate (and Chieko might live another three months), or they could try to get her into an experimental limb sparing program at CSU with Dr. Stephen J. Withrow.

With limb sparing, instead of amputating the limb, ACC surgeons cut away the cancerous tissue, treat the area with chemotherapy, and replace the affected bone with an appropriate-size one from a bank of donor bones. With the help of bone grafts from the patient, the muscles and nerves rearrange themselves using this borrowed piece of skeleton. It's a technically demanding procedure—not for the average orthopedic surgeon, Steve says—but when it succeeds, the animal is up and walking again, suffering only a small decrease in range of motion.

The Herricks brought Chieko to ACC for an evaluation, where she was the comic relief of the waiting room. She'd learned pretty quickly that if she held up her bandaged paw, wounded by her recent biopsy, people would coo in sympathy and might even give her a treat. She had pretty much perfected her pitiful look when she tried it on Steve, who burst out laughing. Steve told them that Chieko would need full-body radiographs to determine if she had cancer anywhere else. If she was accepted into the program, the Herricks would have to pay $1,000, but the research grant would pick up the rest of the cost. If they got Chieko into the program, the result would not be a cure, which happened in only 10 percent of the cases. But it would give them another year or maybe two with Chieko. The Herricks decided to leave Chieko at ACC to be evaluated.

The Herricks drove home in a silence punctuated only by sniffling. A thousand dollars would be tough for the family to come up with. When they pulled into the driveway, Connie raced out of the car, trying to scoop up all of Chieko's toys before Rohn saw them. She had six or seven of them in hand when she started to cry. Signs of Chieko were everywhere—her silly toys, her feeding dishes, the milk bone sticking out of a house plant, the soiled spot on the wallpaper above where she laid, the scratches on the door. If she was accepted, the Herricks decided to use the money they'd saved for new carpeting for Chieko's care. Somehow the old turquoise shag carpet didn't seem quite so bad after all.

Chieko was accepted, and spent Christmas week at ACC undergoing and recovering from the limb-sparing operation. Steve called twice a day over the holidays to let them know how Chieko was doing. Rohn, whose mother was in the hospital with cancer at the same time, was upset that he was getting better service from the veterinarian than he was from his mother's oncologist. "If I ever get cancer," he told Connie, "take me to CSU."

When Chieko returned New Year's Eve, the Herricks slept in sleeping bags next to her on the floor to keep her company. In May 1991, the cancer metastasized and Chieko's right rear leg was amputated. Even with three legs, she took morning runs with Connie. In September, when the cancer spread to her other rear leg, Dr. Withrow told the Herricks it was time to stop. On a beautiful crisp fall day, Steve and some others who had cared for Chieko crowded around her and the Herricks under a cottonwood tree near the hospital to say their good-byes. Amidst an outpouring of love, they administered a drug and Chieko passed. A few months later, when the Herricks got a golden retriever puppy, they named it Withrow in honor of the two and a half years a special doctor and friend had given them with Chieko.

Once again, the Herricks had a puppy that children adored, in particular a neighborhood boy named Pete Knuti. Towheaded and large-boned for his age, Pete even looked a little like Withrow, whom he called "Winthrow." Pete, just like Withrow, was known for his spunk. He loved athletics both as a spectator and as a participant. The fall of his eleventh year, three years after Chieko died, Pete couldn't wait for school to begin because he was on the football team. Pete's mother, Bonnie, was sewing patches on his football uniform on a Friday evening, when she saw the lump on his left leg about the size of a baseball. Pete protested loudly as his mother insisted he go to the doctor to have this looked at, which meant he'd miss the first game.

Pete was diagnosed with Ewing's sarcoma, a form of bone cancer similar to Chieko's osteosarcoma. There's a higher incidence of bone cancer in large dogs and rapidly growing humans, and Pete certainly fit the latter category. He was already very tall for his age and his father, Lee, the high school basketball coach, was six feet, seven inches tall. One theory about these bone cancers is that the disease is in some way related to abnormal cell metabolism in rapidly growing bones. Strenuous activity—such as a St. Bernard puppy or a teenager roughhousing—can cause microfractures during periods of rapid growth, and the microfractures later induce these bone cancers, the theory goes. Pete's doctor, Ross Wilkins, also a neighbor of the Herricks and the Knutis, recommended a new procedure called limb sparing to save Pete's leg. He explained that it had been developed at CSU, and that he had worked closely with a veterinarian named Steve Withrow. Five years later, Chieko's legacy was alive.

Pete had the limb-sparing procedure, and a titanium joint was installed above his knee. After surgery, Pete came home in a wheelchair, and endured chemotherapy every three weeks for nine months. The Herrick and Knuti families drew closer because of "Winthrow." Connie received regular calls from Pete asking if she and "Winthrow" would join his mother and him on their daily walk.

By the time summer came around, Pete had only just finished with chemotherapy, but he was starting to do a lot better. Connie insisted that Pete come to Sky High Hope Camp, a camp for children with cancer, where she had begun volunteering while Chieko was being treated at CSU. Steve and Greg work there every year because, they say, it gives them hope and reenergizes them in their work. A kid who comes one year in a wheelchair shows up the next year walking firmly on two legs. A kid ravaged from chemotherapy returns the next time with a flourishing head of hair. "Cancer is the most curable of all chronic diseases," says Greg. "The camp shows you in the faces of these children the hope and the progress we've made."

Another great thing about the camp is that siblings are welcome. Being the sibling of a very sick child presents stresses and loneliness of its own. So much of the family resources and attention must go to its sickest member, the healthy sibling feels selfish asking for even the most minimal consideration. And the stress on marriages is very high. An overwhelming majority of marriages break up when one of the children gets severely ill. The stress on the sibling, who is not protected from these battles, can be overwhelming.

That year, Pete and his sister, Kristi, attended Sky High Hope Camp and met Steve Withrow. The last full day of camp is a beach party, the highlight of which is the canoe races for the coveted "Styrofoam Cup" trophy. Pete asked Steve to be his partner in the race and they won, with Connie Herrick and Greg Ogilvie standing on the shore cheering them on. "Here was the man who had made limb sparing possible for kids, and there was one of those kids in a canoe race with him," Connie said.

Besides being winning canoe partners, Steve and Pete became friends. Pete's father, Lee, says that, while the two were different in style, they were equally intense. When Pete had to shadow someone for career day, he chose Steve, and even spent the night at his house. And for three years straight they took the Styrofoam Cup. On Christmas Eve 1997, five years after Pete's original diagnosis, he was diagnosed with leukemia, which is a side effect of the chemotherapy in 2 percent of cases. Steve called Pete as soon as he heard the diagnosis. He drove to Denver to watch the NFL playoffs with Pete, and after that came to visit every week.

Pete was scheduled for a bone marrow transplant when he developed an infection in his leg that the doctors were unable to clear up. An amputation was scheduled before the transplant. On the morning of the amputation, Steve called Pete to wish him luck. Then Steve went to a tattoo parlor—armed with his own needles and dye—and had a tattoo of a cancer crab with the circle and slash denoting "no" on top of it. At the bottom were the initials, P. K. He sent a fax of the tattoo to Pete on which he wrote: "It hurt like hell, but not as much as your amputation."

Pete next had the bone marrow transplant and did very well. It seemed as though Pete had beaten the odds. On St. Patrick's Day, Pete returned home and the whole neighborhood turned out to welcome him. His recovery had truly been a community project. The neighbors had run a blood drive—the largest blood drive that Bonfils Blood Bank had had in a single day—and sold T-shirts that read "For Pete's Sake . . . and others, too!" Kristi, then a sophomore at Harvard, flew home every weekend on frequent flyer miles donated by her neighbors. Neighbors had made meals for the family, house-sat while they were at the hospital, and even did their laundry.

But Pete's stay at home was cut short. He was back in the hospital in April 1998, where he died shortly before Easter. His memorial service was attended by more than a thousand people, with an overflowing crowd in the school cafeteria who listened to the service on an audio feed. Steve Withrow came, but didn't speak to the crowd. He still has the Styrofoam Cup with their winning times displayed proudly in his office at ACC. Kristi, who did her honors thesis on Sky High Hope Camp, has been accepted to medical school at the University of Colorado, where she intends to study pediatric oncology.

Ten years later, the legacy of Chieko and the other dogs treated under the research protocol at ACC is still alive. When Dr. Ross Wilkins and Dr. Steve Withrow began working together on bone cancer in 1986, others thought their quest was pointless. The course of treatment was to immediately amputate the limb, because by the time doctors detected the disease, the cancer in most cases had already metastasized. Eighty percent of the patients had amputations, yet despite this, 80 percent of them died.

Working together, Steve and Ross experimented with delivering che-motherapy through the artery that feeds the cancer so that a strong dose can go directly to the tumor. They strengthened the donor bones with a bone cement mixed with antibiotics to fight infection, and they pio-neered culturing growth factors from donor tissue to stimulate the body to accept the new bone. Now, sixteen years later, 90 percent of patients keep their limbs, and 80 percent of them survive.

When people say they are fighting cancer, a lot of what they are fighting is the debilitating fear and loneliness of a diagnosis that feels like a death sentence. As with so many experiences with our animals, when you have your pet alongside you, you not only don't feel so alone, you feel alive. Loved. Needed. Bill Johnson teaming up with Max to fight cancer is, these stories show, a microcosm of the larger experience that many people have with pets and cancer, whether the pet is the one with the diagnosis, or the human is.

The medical breakthroughs ricochet from animal to human and back to animal again, as in Bill's uncanny victory of getting a top Mayo Clinic radiologist to look at his dog's cancer. For the Herricks and Chieko, the expenditure of money wasn't nearly as extravagant as Bill Johnson's, but it was more difficult for them to come up with their $1,000. The beauty of the way this reflects the Bond is how both sides benefit not just from the medical advances, but from the uniting in spirit against a common foe. The fight against cancer then becomes not just researchers working in the laboratories and families struggling alone with their pain and fear, but a cause for neighbors to rally round, as it became in Wheat Ridge, where one dog and one child's illness touched so many lives. And the rookie volunteers at Sky High Hope Camp are Mike Lingenfelter and Dakota, joined by my son, Lex, and I.

The new way researchers are putting animals to use in the fight against cancer is by using them for early detection. Dermatologist Dr. Armand Cognetta practices in Tallahassee, smack in the middle of the Florida Sunbelt, a practice in which melanomas are more common than Micky Mouse ears.

After a particularly grinding few months, months during which he'd detected more than a hundred melanomas with his handheld microscope, Dr. Cognetta began to wonder if he couldn't come up with a better method for early detection. He was driving home from work one night when he heard Paul Harvey on the radio talking about cops who were trying to find a body at the bottom of a lake. Instead of dredging, they were using a dog, who stood at the prow of the boat sniffing the air. Dr. Cognetta found this remarkable. If a dog could detect a body at the bottom of the lake twenty or thirty feet underwater, he'd bet one could be trained to sniff out melanoma. He set out to find a trainer willing to work on this idea.

He found Duane Pickel, a man who has worked his whole life training dogs to sniff out anomalies. When Duane was in Vietnam, he trained dogs as scouts. He and his dog would crawl on their bellies in the tall grass looking for snipers in the trees. Duane had his companion on a short leash—less than a yard long—and the two would leapfrog silently forward. If the dog spotted someone, Duane would feel the dog's throat rumbling on the leash before the growl was audible. The points of his raised ears perfectly framed the location of the sniper.

When he got home, Duane trained bomb-sniffing dogs for the first President Bush, and spent twenty years as a canine officer in the Tallahassee Police Department. Duane says he literally cannot count the number of times his life has been saved by the keen senses of his canine pals. "I find dogs to be smarter than eighty percent of the people I work with, and all the people I work for," he says.

A dog's sense of smell for some odors is ten million times more acute than ours. Humans have five to fifteen million receptors in the nose devoted to smell, and dogs have two hundred and fifty million, says Dr. Jim Walker, director of the Sensory Research Institute in Florida. So confident is Duane of a dog's olfactory skills that he believes he can train a dog to detect anything that is different from its surrounding environment. So although he'd been working most of his life on bombs and drugs, Duane was eager for the melanoma challenge. He had just the dog to do it—George.

George was a standard schnauzer, whom Duane chose for his intelligence, superior bloodline, and small size. He wanted a smaller-size dog than the traditional bomb-sniffing and drug-detecting dog because he wanted a canine that could crawl into tight spaces in airplanes in search of bombs. By the time Dr. Cognetta's challenge came along, George had more than proven his olfactory skills. He had six American Kennel Club titles, two obedience trial championships, four world records, and four hundred first places in competition. At the United States Police Canine competition, George was the only dog in the history of the event to find forty-seven out of forty-seven bombs in a week's worth of trials.

Dr. Cognetta provided Duane with tumor samples, which he placed in test tubes. He trained George to distinguish the smell of melanoma from the smell of benign cancers and samples of noncancerous skin. He had the samples in a test tube rack. When George detected cancer, he'd do a passive alert—just sit still. Duane would then ask him: "Show me." George would nudge the test tube with his nose. When Duane asked again for George to show him, George would lay his paw on top of the test tube. George got up to a 99 percent accuracy rate, so they decided to test him on humans.

Dr. Cognetta got several brave souls to volunteer to be sniffed by George. The pictures Duane has from this experiment in progress really make you smile at what you can get people to do. Several people lay on the floor in their bathing suits with different kinds of tumor samples taped to their bodies with Band-Aids. Then Duane let George loose to sniff every crevice. He found every single one of the cancerous tumors and none of the false samples. When Dr. Cognetta found a few brave patients willing to let George have a sniff of bare skin, he found six melanomas undetectable by a handheld microscope.

"The dog is smelling something, and what he's smelling is unique to melanoma," says Dr. Walker. Walker was so intrigued by George's success that he and his wife and research partner, Dianne Beidler Walker, are working with Duane to take the research the next step further.

George died late in 2000, so Dianne and Duane are training another schnauzer named Stormy to replace him. They are also working to identify the exact chemical marker that the dog detects by analyzing the molecules that float in the air, or head space, above the melanoma samples. Once Stormy is trained and the marker she detects is identified, it may be possible to build a machine that can smell melanoma. Some people would still rather have a dog, however. "We've had families with high risk of melanoma *beg* to have a dog sniff them," Dianne notes.

Nancy Best believes dogs can sniff out cancer because her golden Lab, Mia, found her breast cancer in time to save her life. At age thirty-nine, Nancy had been having health problems for a number of years and had seen a lot of doctors, each of whom tried to deal with the specific symptom. None of them got a holistic perspective on Nancy's chronic full-body pain, fatigue, insomnia, weight gain, and depression. In 1998, just a few months before Nancy was diagnosed with fibromyalgia, she got a golden Labrador retreiver she named Mia.

She named her Mia because she wanted a dog who was wholly and completely hers. She'd had many animals all her life. She and her husband and three kids have quite a menagerie on the land they own in Garberville, the gateway to California's redwood forests: a cat, two parrots, several exotic chickens to which Mia made a great addition. It was a time of great promise in Nancy's life, despite her physical complaints. The coffee cart business she'd started in front of a gas station in 1993 had gradually expanded into a coffeehouse named the Java Joint. In August 1999, Nancy had opened a full-fledged nightclub in an old bank building with coffee and pastries early in the morning, and live music and a full bar at night. Suddenly, shortly after the grand opening, Nancy noticed that Mia was acting oddly.

Nancy came home every afternoon for an hour-and-a-half nap before her daughter got home from school. Usually Nancy lay on the couch with Mia at her side. In September, four months after Nancy's negative mammogram, Mia wouldn't leave Nancy's shirt alone. She kept sniffing and licking at Nancy's right breast. When Mia continued the behavior for the third day in a row, Nancy put her outside. Otherwise, Nancy wouldn't be able to get in her nap.

That afternoon when her daughter opened the screen door, Mia bolted through the door and dived right at that same spot at Nancy's right breast. The spot hurt terribly from Mia's pressure, much more so than the normal amount of chronic pain from fibromyalgia. Nancy touched the spot and felt a mass. It was a Type 2 estrogen-positive invasive ductal carcinoma, an extremely fast-growing cancer that, if not detected early, can kill a woman in six months. Having just had a negative mammogram, and with no familial history of cancer, Nancy would never have been looking for cancer. "Mia knew it and she made sure I knew it, too," Nancy said. "Without her, I would have died." Nancy's doctor, Mark Phelps, agrees. "We need to learn to pay attention to our world and appreciate the keen senses dogs have," he said. "When we're sick, we should not only listen to our bodies, but listen to our pets."

Nancy sold her business immediately, only one month after she'd gotten her dream up and running, because she had to concentrate full-time on getting well. When she sold the Java Joint, she decided to reward herself by buying a two-carat diamond ring from a local jeweler for $17,000. She drove by the Java Joint every day and wanted to be able to look down at the ring she called "the healing stone" and say, "I don't have the business, but I have this." After only a few weeks, the magic wore off of the ring. It didn't bring her health and happiness. She sold it back to the jeweler and bought an African Grey parrot she named Ruby because of its big red tail. Ruby brought her love and laughter, a diamond in the rough that she could train.

She underwent four months of radiation, a partial mastectomy, and the most aggressive chemotherapy her body could endure. "My hair fell out in fourteen days," she recalls. Although she's cancer-free in her right breast, she has to be checked every three months for the next five years to make sure there's no recurrence.

It's been a very tough three years for Nancy, years she's sure she'd not have survived without Mia. Most of her days are dominated with managing the pain of fibromyalgia, a condition that is invisible to most people outside her family. "Sometimes I feel like I should wear a number on my chest so that people will know what level of pain I'm enduring," she said. "But Mia always knows when something is wrong."

"Any time that you have an emotional or biological change, there's a chemical change in your body, and your dog can detect it," Duane Pickel says. "They detect something in you because they love you and you're a member of their pack. But it's a whole different ball game from that dog looking for cancer in somebody else."

Although the results are similar, in that both George and Mia detected cancer, the point of connection is opposite. Duane Pickel comes at the problem like a detective who is looking for a new tool for his arsenal.

He wants to train a high-performing obedience dog to use his acute sense of smell as a fail-safe device to sniff out cancer in anyone. It's actually a challenge that goes beyond the specifics of cancer for Duane, who believes in his heart that humans have only started to employ the amazing power of animals' senses for human benefit. He cites the dogs that work the Alaskan oil pipeline, whose noses can detect one part natural gas in one trillion parts air.

What Nancy has in Mia is something similar to what Dakota has with Mike—another creature that watches so closely that he or she can detect the slightest variation in humor, either physical or mental. That's a different kind of expectation from what Duane has and one more closely linked to the major service animals provide to cancer patients—a sense that in this time of hopelessness, they don't really have to be alone.

Jack Stephens, who founded and runs Veterinary Pet Insurance, is a veterinarian who's been a friend of mine for almost twenty years. He's a rugged outdoorsman, a tough Oklahoma cowboy who favored the larger breeds of dogs for hunting, and was unsentimental about the relationship between man and beast. For many years, I'd see Jack all but roll his eyes when I'd launch into one of my reveries about the Bond. Of course, Jack is a pet lover and has had animals around him all his life. But when his clients would burst into tears when their dog got sick or when they described annoying acts as if they were endearing traits, Jack had to discipline himself not to tell them what he thought of all this "canine nonsense."

In 1989, Jack was diagnosed with Stage 4 throat cancer. "At the time I thought there must be ten or twelve levels," Jack said. "I didn't know four was the top, as grim as it could get. They gave me only six months to a year to live." The affected area is a pretty tight space, and radiation could damage a lot of the delicate tissue around the tumor. His doctors proposed removing his tongue and his jawbone. "What would be the point?" Jack thought. "I wouldn't be able to eat or talk. It wouldn't have been a very good life at all."

A few months before his diagnosis, Jack's wife, Vicki, got a miniature Doberman pinscher, Spanky, who initially annoyed Jack. He hated little dogs. He found something about them undignified. "It's not manly to have a little dog," he said. "And they don't have a purpose." But Spanky endeared himself to Jack because of his expressive face and pugnacious personality. Spanky had definite ideas about how he wanted to be treated. He didn't like to be left alone. Frequently when the Stephens left him at home, they'd come back to find he'd expressed his displeasure by toilet-papering the house like some teenage Halloween prank. For some reason, despite Jack's gruffness, Spanky was really drawn to him. And even more so when Jack came down with cancer.

He followed Jack everywhere, lying on his lap when he sat, on the headrest behind him when he drove, and with his head on the pillow alongside Jack when he went to sleep at night. In this time of need, Jack's prejudice about small, clingy dogs crumbled. "It took me a while to get over having him with me out in public, but not very long, though. I used to think people were crazy who took their dogs everywhere with them, like the animal didn't know his place," Jack said. "Then I started taking him to the grocery store, to the hardware store, and talking to him all the time. He seemed to sense my moods and my needs and was very, very attentive and affectionate."

When Jack went in for radiation treatments, he brought Spanky along. In the long sleepless nights that followed, Spanky was his constant companion. "Sometimes I'd be real sick afterward and he knew when, where, and how to approach," Jack said. When Jack was at his lowest, Spanky would get right into his arms and demand to be petted. Other times he'd stay three feet away, knowing that Jack didn't really want someone close. He'd also make Jack exercise. "He'd go to the front door and jump and jump until I took him out," Jack said. "If he hadn't done that, I would have just sat around feeling sorry for myself. That is the downward spiral of cancer that I think that pets definitely help you overcome." As an honor to Spanky and Skeeter, a miniature Doberman who succeeded him, Jack has established the Skeeter Foundation, which grants money to researchers investigating the healing power of pets.

The powerful effect a pet has in breaking the downward spiral of cancer patients is something Dr. Edward T. Creagan, oncology professor at the Mayo Medical School, has seen repeatedly in his own practice. He's such a strong believer in the ability of pets to ameliorate the devastating emotional impact of a cancer diagnosis that he suggests that the patient acquire a pet in a third of his cases.

He first noticed how important pets were to his patients ten years ago when he was consulting with a woman who had Stage 4 lung cancer. The topic switched to Reggie, and the woman became almost buoyant in talking about this creature whom Dr. Creagan assumed was her husband. As the conversation continued, he realized Reggie was her cat.

"I became fascinated by the conversation about pets, which defused the anguish and the suffering of cancer," Dr. Creagan says. "Pets are a conduit for wellness. This woman was not a recluse, like so many patients become. To care for Reggie, she had to buy cat food and take Reggie to the vet. That sort of physical activity buoyed the spirits."

Dr. Creagan started making a point of writing the names of the patients' pets on their charts and asking about them at each appointment. "There is a lightness, an element of levity in recognizing the pet that defuses some of the angst of the encounter," he believes. The effect of giving love to a pet, Dr. Creagan says, creates a positive self-image of caring at a time when the patient is increasingly dependent. "I think it creates healing of the soul. Some of the anger and the resentment is channeled in a positive way for caring for the pet."

The most important benefit Dr. Larry Lachman, a Carmel, California, psychologist, believes pets provide to cancer patients is their ability to listen without judgment. Dr. Lachman, who has survived prostate cancer with the help of his flat-coated retriever, Max, believes the primary way someone suffering from a chronic illness deals with their trauma is by talking about it, something Dr. Lachman calls the "illness narrative."

"Even relatives and family members can only take so much of their emotions," Dr. Lachman said. "Pets don't mind hearing the traumas of the illness narrative over and over. It helps the patient get over the post-traumatic stress of illness and treatment."

One of the many traumas of getting cancer is how much fear you inspire in others. Even the most well-meaning friends frequently touch a cancer patient gingerly, as if they are afraid that the cancer was contagious. That unspoken horror affects the patient deeply. While undergoing treatment, Dr. Lachman found himself shying away from the touch he craved. "With so much surgical touch and medical touch, I recoiled. I was conditioned to expect pain," he said. "But animals give permission to touch and be touched. So Max and my massage therapist desensitized me and retaught my body on a visceral level that touch is not always traumatic."

Pets also have a remarkable sixth sense to perceive and cognate, long before an actual signal is sent or received, to know what's coming or to alert to a danger. On a challenge from a behaviorist, I observed my dogs sleeping both in the house and outside the house over the period of several weeks. Routinely, even when I looked through the window at Sirloin or LLLucky lying on the grass twenty feet away, sleeping dogs wouldn't lie as they would alert to my glance and get up or lift their heads in the canine version of "Whazzzzzuuuuuuup!" This uncanny sixth sense also works when a pet seems to know that you've had a bad-hair day or a no-hair day from the last round of chemotherapy or are coming home early from work and the dog runs to the door when you are still miles from home.

Our animal companions can detect the low mood of illness, the need for play, and distraction from our woes. Is it any wonder, then, that humans try in the limited ways they can to honor the Bond by sacrificing time and money—in some cases, careers—to save their precious pals from the scariest disease, cancer? In this disease, the benefits of the Bond clearly flow both ways, working to strengthen the health and well-being of all.

Chronic Pain—Take Two Pets and Call Me in the Morning

MY OLDER BROTHER BOB INHERITED our father's name, and with it his perfectionism. Bob left the farm as soon as he finished high school and became a corporate lawyer with a much bigger territory to scrutinize than a farm. I'm sure his sharp eye for imperfection served him well in business, but it made him hard to be around at family gatherings, usually the only time we'd see each other, as we live on opposite ends of the state. The family joke was that Bob suffered from motion sickness, the uncontrollable desire to leave before he even reached his destination. While he stayed, his head swiveled to every movement or sound, and I often noticed him grinding his teeth while he listened. Sometimes being in a room with him reminded me of the jars of fruit in my mother's old pressure cooker as it slowly built to a boil.

One morning in April of 1998, Bob woke up to bilateral numbness in his limbs and shortly thereafter was diagnosed with multiple sclerosis. Bob and his family traveled extensively in search of a cure and conferred with many specialists, but he got no relief. Bob's condition worsened quickly. He lost part of his vision and hearing, and started to suffer constant pain in his legs that did not respond to drugs, massage, even the laying on of hands by his church family.

He tried valiantly to maintain a life as close as he could to what it had been before he got sick. On the first summer after his diagnosis, he and his family went on their annual fishing trip to Stanley, Idaho, where they had rented the same cabin on the banks of the Salmon River for more than a decade. But on this trip, Bob found the banks too steep and slippery for his unsteady legs. He watched from a distance as his wife, Lisa, and boys, Sam and Joe, fished their favorite hole. By 2000, Bob's condition had deteriorated so much that they didn't even bother to make a reservation. On the phone, his voice was frequently a halting, low monotone, his strong façade on the verge of crumbling. Sometimes I'd feel so futile and stupid trying to cheer him up, like trying to tape a happy face over a mask of pain. I would tell him there were miracles and that he needed to release the worry to God. Let Him worry about this, I said, and focus on the things you are still able to do.

Our mom told me that Bob was having a particularly dark week. A respected physician had given hope of another miracle cure, only to have it fall far short of the promise. When I called, rather than trying to preach about keeping his spirits up, I tried a new tactic. We're always telling ailing loved ones to appreciate the moment, but every question we ask encourages them to describe their hopelessness so we can offer sympathy. I decided to ask him a question that would bring him into the moment: "When do you feel the very best?"

"I feel the best when I come home from work, or just come in from the next room and Buddy rushes to greet me," he said brightly, referring to the Yorkshire terrier he'd gotten less than a year before. "I sit in the chair and Buddy jumps up on my lap, where his body soothes my legs. Then he washes my feet and knees with a thousand licks. I really love that. Marty, you've got to meet him."

Here I was thinking he was going to say that wrapping his aching legs in an electric blanket or getting a massage from Lisa was the time he felt the best. Or maybe it was when the new pain pills or his high-tech morphine pump kicked in. I have to admit that when people who suffer chronic pain say that the thing that helps the most is their pet, I can see it, I can feel it, I believe it, but I don't understand how it works.

For example, my wife, Teresa, has rheumatoid arthritis, and there are some mornings when it's difficult for her to get out of bed. Thanks to medication and motivation, she always finds a way. She says she has to, for the dogs. I know when Teresa has entered the kitchen by the furious, scrambling sound of Scooter, as she scampers over the floor toward the pet pantry (formerly our pantry), her feet tap-dancing across the hardwood floor like the world's only four-legged Rockette, and certainly the only one with a beard.

In a sickeningly sweet, high-pitched voice, Teresa asks Scooter which one of the treats she'd like. Scooter indicates her preference by clawing at Teresa's leg like some canine Freddy Krueger. Teresa claims she always knows which treat Scooter is going to pick. Each morning, she repeats her question, then pets Scooter as she eats. But with LLLucky the ritual is a lot quieter. As LLLucky eats his food, she gently, rhythmically strokes his body from the tip of his nose to the tip of his tail. When we first adopted him from an abusive home, his horrific past had made him suspicious. He'd only eat when Teresa was petting him. He's relaxed a lot over the past year, but Teresa still pets him while he eats and, on mornings when her joints are particularly achy, the petting continues long after the meal is through.

When you're in pain, you want something, anything that works, and you're willing to explore drug-free remedies that often get overlooked by physicians. You know that the agony of chronic pain is not "all in your head," but experts say that much of the means for coping with it may be.

Many studies of the ways pets help with chronic conditions point to how they stimulate routine as one of their benefits. For people who need to take pills several times a day or those who must really watch their eating, the low hum of activity needed to care for a pet creates an underlying structure on which the human can hang the new tasks. Teresa has things that she must do every day, and doing them makes pain the aberration. "Acting like Valium, but with no side effects, pets have a powerful anxiolytic effect that lowers the pain threshold," says Virginia Byers-Kraus, M.D., Ph.D., a rheumatologist and associate professor of medicine at Duke University School of Medicine. "Plus studies show that people with severe arthritis move even less than sedentary people. I find that patients will often do for a pet what they won't do for themselves. Pets bring activity, and from activity springs health."

The newest thinking on the treatment of pain addresses what doctors call palliative care. To palliate (from the Latin word *palliare*, which means "to cloak") is to make something seem less severe and intense. Dr. Ann Berger, who heads up pain and palliative care at the National Institutes of Health, divides pain into two parts: the pain itself and the larger component suffering, which amplifies the perception of pain. As Ann points out, there is no way to measure the amount of pain a person is in. "Pain is really whatever a person says it is," she says. "We don't have MRIs or CAT scans like we do for other things to measure pain. The suffering part of pain is the emotional side of illness: fear of loss of work, disability, isolation, and spiritual concerns. The suffering is never helped with just medicine."

Ann cited the example of a person who comes into the doctor complaining of a cough. The doctor does a "multimillion-dollar workup" and diagnoses lung cancer. "So a whole treatment plan is made up of chemo, radiation, plus or minus surgery, but nobody looks at the whole person," Ann said. "That's how we've always functioned in medicine. Yes, we want to cure the cancer. But we also want to make an attempt at curing the person."

Outside her office at the NIH stands a teacart with a silver tea service, fine china cups, and several boxes of expensive European cookies. Draped across the handles of the cart are wigs, big silly hats, scarves, and bright feather boas. Patients whose treatments have caused them to lose their hair can wear these when Ann comes to serve them high tea at 3:00 P.M. She also uses music and art therapy, tai chi, acupuncture, biofeedback, counseling, and spiritual care. But one of her favorite tools is pets.

Patients come from all over the country and the world to participate in government-funded medical research at the National Institutes of Health, the nation's premier research hospital just north of Washington, D.C., in Bethesda, Maryland. Many of them have been sick for a long time, and face lengthy hospital stays cut off from their families, making it even harder for them to maintain an identity beyond just being a collection of symptoms and reams of test results. Mondays and Thursdays, when animal assisted therapy teams from Capital Canines come to NIH, Ann draws up a list of patients she thinks could benefit from a visit.

The night I visited, I walked with a team to see a teenager who was spending his junior year of high school at NIH for treatment of a severe gastric condition. When we came to the door of his room, he had the lights off and the television on and he told us he didn't want to see anyone. The teams travel with a recreational therapist, who insisted that he let in M.G., a cute little shih tzu. The young man had something like sixty-two staples up and down the side of his body, and was stiff with the pain and the loneliness. M.G. has been trained to crawl low to the bed on his belly, under the covers even, to get as close to the ailing patient as he can. With the canine comforter pressed gently up against the incision, you could see this guy relax. His hand found the dog and he started to stroke him. Just then the phone rang, and he said, "I can't talk to you right now, there's a dog here," and hung up to continue stroking the dog. It was astonishing to see this wall crumble because of the strength of the Bond.

The emotional component of this brief exchange between the teenager and M.G. is so clear. At a time when most of this young man's peers have a near heart attack about getting a pimple and agonize over exactly which T-shirt is best for which occasion, he had come to think of tubes and wires as his apparel. His illness had caused a huge strain on the family, and visits from his relatives had become awkward. His parents were having problems, and he was beginning to think those were his fault. But M.G. knew nothing about any of that. He just sensed a kid in pain, and was drawn to help.

What is less apparent is the powerful, life-enhancing chemicals the time with M.G. releases in the young man's brain. Many of our feelings, thoughts, and attitudes are influenced by changes in brain chemistry. Biochemicals such as phenylethalamine (amphetaminelike), dopamine, beta-endorphin, prolactin, and oxytocin are natural substances that increase in the bloodstream when bonding takes place and stimulate feelings of elation, safety, tranquility, happiness, satisfaction, nurturing, even love.

When South African Prof. Johannes Odendaal studied the physiological basis for the effectiveness of animal assisted therapy, he wanted to see how long the human needed to interact with the pet before the benefits of the contact between them could be recorded. In his experiment, he allowed people to stroke, touch, and talk softly to well-mannered dogs, either their own or a stranger's, while he monitored their blood pressure. After the pairs had settled down for ten minutes, he attached a continuous blood pressure monitor to both pet and human.

When blood pressure dropped 5 to 10 percent, as it did for both species in about ten minutes, Odendaal drew blood from both. He went beyond previous tests that measured triglycerides and cholesterol and tested for the presence of mood-altering biochemicals.

Analysis of the blood revealed that the positive biochemicals increased significantly for both the pets and people. The humans who were interacting with their own dogs had even higher elevations of these chemicals in their blood, demonstrating more powerful positive effects of the Bond beyond the simple contact. Odendaal concluded that he had "uncovered a physiological reason to attempt to establish . . . such positive interaction." Just like amphetamines shouldn't be a substitute for pursuing natural pleasure or excitement, pets shouldn't be used to exclude the bond between humans. But just when they're needed most, pets are powerful drugs indeed.

I've witnessed firsthand that when Teresa pets LLLucky, she relaxes, mind, body, and soul. Study after study proves that the simple act of petting the dogs drops Teresa's blood pressure and makes her pulse deeper and slower with the rhythm of her strokes. Nearly identical to what happens when a mother nurses a child, a human petting a dog feels safe, nurturing, and at home. She is at peace with her animal nature, and she needn't think about the worries of the day or her aching joints. More important for the Bond, as she strokes LLLucky, the Odendaal study shows, hormones and neuropeptides bathe both of their nervous systems. Through this simple, soothing motion, the destructive duo of stress—adrenaline and cortisone—are body-slammed, as is the suffering. As Dr. Ann Berger says: "Suffering is where we need the non-pharmacological things."

Just stroking LLLucky isn't going to cure Teresa's arthritis; that's clear. Taking medicine for it doesn't cure it, either; it just suppresses the symptoms and dulls the pain. Both factors—the Bond and her medicines—are helping Teresa to live a productive life despite her illness. I wouldn't want to risk a reversal in her health by taking either away.

The Odendaal study also demonstrates that pets offer a benefit to those who don't own animals and don't even want one. When a champagne-colored kitten appeared on Sharon Weisswasser's doorstep wearing a "please give me a home" message on his collar, she just wanted it to go away. She didn't really like cats, and had bought a dog two years ago to help with her pain from multiple sclerosis. When she found the cat, Sharon was at the lowest point since she was diagnosed at age eighteen. She'd had to resign her position as the manager of an accounting firm because the vision problems and fatigue of multiple sclerosis had made it impossible to continue working. Before her kids and she could find a new owner for the stray kitty, she fell for Gato, who made such a great companion for her chocolate Lab. She loved watching them curled up together on the couch.

Gato curled up with Sharon, too. The beta injections she was receiving gave her flulike symptoms and plunged her into depression. When her fever spiked to 106 degrees, he was right at her side. All she could do was stare out the window all day, but the animals, particularly Gato, never left her. Gato, who with Sharon was featured in the 2001 National Multiple Sclerosis Society "Pet Power" calendar, has never weighed more than seven pounds, and still likes to be cradled in Sharon's arms like a baby. "When you can sit there and hold him like a baby," Sharon said, "it has a healing effect. You can't fight the healing power of the animal right up against you. Your body can't reject it."

Part of chronic pain is structural, says Dr. Jeff Burgess, an attending physician at the University of Washington Pain Center. Bones, muscles, joints, and nerves can serve as sources of raw pain. As chronic pain builds, normal activity grinds to a halt. Lethargy is often followed by anxiety and depression. "Pets can make people more relaxed, elevate their mood, and keep them moving," Dr. Burgess says.

For people with arthritis, which now affects nearly 43 million Americans, "movement" is the movement. "We've come from thinking that physical fitness was impossible for people with arthritis, to knowing that exercise is one of the best ways to manage their disease and minimize their disability," says Marian Minor, a physical therapy professor at the University of Missouri–Columbia and codirector of the Arthritis Rehabilitation Research and Training Center. In this way, the effect of animals is as much physical therapy as it is treatment for the suffering. "Pets provide meaningful activity and energize people who are often thinking, Should I get up or sit here?" Dr. Minor said.

Joan Neely, who has suffered with rheumatoid arthritis for twenty years, uses her bay gelding horse, Chinook, to keep her joints limber. She boards Chinook at a stable with an indoor arena so they can work at dressage three to four times a week, even when the Spokane winters get harsh. She's grateful that Chinook is so patient with her because they've been doing the same course work for almost five years with only marginal improvement. "He can do lead changes, but not when I ask for them," Joan says, assessing the sorry state of their efforts. "And our canter and our pirouettes are not very good. He'd be much better if he had a better rider."

In order to make the horse do what she needs it to do for dressage, she has to be soft and flexible. "In dressage, you are judged by the quality of your gait," Joan said. "If you are stiff, the horse's walk will be very stilted." Chinook helps her to fight an arthritis sufferer's tendency to protect her shoulders and spine. "You have to be very flexible in the spine. The arms have to follow the bit, so the arms have to be flexible beginning with the shoulders. It took me five years to relax my shoulders, just to know how to feel them."

The effect of this therapy lasts into the next day for Joan, and when she goes on vacation or misses more than a few sessions, she has to learn to let go of the tension there all over again. The other ripple effect of working with the horse is the sensory stimulation of the way the horse feels and smells, Joan said, and the concentration it takes to make the horse move the way you want it to go. "When you are concentrating on the horse, you take your mind off your body. Whatever it is you want to accomplish with the horse has to come through your body to the horse," she observed. "There is a real sense of accomplishment when you make that connection, knowing that, especially for a person with arthritis, you got your mind and body to move as one."

Dr. Meredith Heick, Joan's rheumatologist in Spokane, Washington, says that most of her patients are struggling just to continue the basic activities of daily living. She is proud that Joan has taken on a sport that demands physical and technical skill. "Joan's being able to compete and improve in a demanding sport such as dressage has a relaxational effect and a big mental payoff that, taken together, moderates the severity of her arthritis," Dr. Heick said.

"Pets may help people in two major ways," says Dr. Burgess. "By initiating and maintaining the relaxation response, pets can take people's focus off of their pain and elevate their moods. Secondly, through touch or physical contact, they can block the transmission of their pain from the periphery to the central nervous system, shutting the pain-processing centers down." He mentioned a recent article in the research journal *Pain* that featured a PET (positron emission tomography) scan of a person using a counterirritant to block pain. It showed a reduced blood flow and reduced activities in these areas; a high-tech confirmation of sorts for what many patients have been feeling and saying for years: hypnosis and other nontraditional therapies such as pets work. Although Dr. Burgess was talking specifically about the act of petting an animal, clearly for many sufferers of chronic pain, the distraction effect is broadened by any time people spend focusing attention away from their pain and onto their pets.

Equally important is the attention that pets lavish on their human companions. Many people, not just those who suffer from chronic pain, mention how their animals know just when they are hurting and how to draw just close enough to help soothe those feelings. The notion that this creature is unafraid to be with you in this dark time is very comforting.

Judy McDonough has been very sick for a very long time. She was diagnosed with juvenile onset diabetes when she was only ten years old, and had managed to keep that pretty much under control. She had always rescued wildlife, volunteering at animal shelters since she was sixteen. At age twenty-three, she was working toward a degree in wildlife rehabilitation at my alma mater, Washington State University, when she came down with rheumatoid arthritis. As her symptoms increased in severity, she had to quit school, but she continued to volunteer at the wildlife rehabilitation clinic because she got so much out of working with the animals. She was particularly fond of a completely blind barn owl that she and her colleagues had named Stevie Wonder because of the distinct way he bobbed his head.

Ten years ago, she had to quit that part-time job because the pain in her joints was so severe. Since then, she's accumulated her own palliative care staff in the form of her Italian greyhound, Emma; her mixed breed dog, Meghan; and her one-eyed alley cat, Elliot.

Both Emma and Elliot are highly attuned to Judy's bouts of suffering. When Judy is having such a bad day that she dozes off to sleep on the couch, when she wakes up she'll find that Emma has lined up her five favorite toys next to Judy. It's an offering of concern, Judy believes, because it's not done with a wag and a jump to indicate that it's time to play. Emma moves the toys there so quietly that she never wakes Judy up.

Elliot and she have a special link based on the way he came into

Judy's life. A friend found Elliot in an alleyway with his jaw cracked, his nose broken, and a severely damaged right eye. Judy rushed him into surgery, where they repaired most of his face, but could not save the eye. Ever since he came home from the hospital, Elliot has demonstrated his gratitude by his intense loyalty to Judy. At times when she's really struggling with the competing side effects of her arthritis medicines as well as the drugs she takes for diabetes, she describes herself as being in "survival mode." It's hard to even think of getting out of bed. "On those days, Elliot will come beside me and lay his leg on my arm. He only does that when I'm in really bad shape," Judy says. "My friend who found him calls him my little angel. He's a very peaceful cat for all he's been through."

The touch of the cat and the gifts of the dog all serve as relaxants for Judy, who says she manages to stay pretty positive most of the time because of her friends, her spirituality, and her pets. "They redirect me when I'm depressed," Judy said. "They are so easy to be around. They don't take any of your energy away. When everything gets so complicated, they are so simple. I know I can get through with their unconditional love." "With depression, pain is always a more significant component of daily life," says Dr. Joseph Waters, our family physician in Twin Falls. "What I see with my patients is that with pets, pain can become a nonentity." A nonentity?

After talking to pain specialists about how this pet prescription for pain could actually work, I wanted to see my brother Bob's magical Yorkie, Buddy. Having just visited the family gravesite in Buhl, Idaho, family totems and symbols were fresh on my mind. The Becker "one bar one, or spread H" brand graced my grandfather and grandmother's tombstone, and had as much meaning to us as a family crest. I was delighted as I pulled into my brother Bob's driveway for the first visit in two years and saw a ONE BAR ONE RANCH sign swinging on the archway.

I hugged Bob at the door and as I moved over the threshold, I followed his pointing finger down, way down, to see a wild frenzy of welcome. Buddy was spinning cartwheels at my feet and raking the air with his front legs like a miniature stallion. As I knelt down for a closer look, Buddy launched himself into my lap and began machine-gunning kisses onto every patch of skin he could find.

Like a parent preparing his child for class pictures, Bob had just had Buddy groomed, and I admired the steel-blue hair on his body and vibrating tail and the chestnut-colored tan of his face and feet. Buddy's ears were erect like two perfect triangles positioned high on his head, and his open mouth showed teeth that were Ultra Brite white. A spirited and sparking character, the most defining characteristic of Buddy was his eyes. Being a veterinarian, I've seen hundreds of Yorkies in my twenty-year-plus career, but I'd never seen any dog with more expressive eyes than Buddy. They were the size of small dewy grapes, dark and reflective, sparkling with intelligence and an almost uncanny look of understanding.

I got Buddy to sit in the crook of my crossed legs. I started rubbing the full length of his stomach in an Aladdin lamp move, and soon his right rear foot was scratching the air in slow motion. I looked into the center of his eyes, cooing, "You're a goooooood boy, Buddy, I love you," and moved from his belly to rubbing the inside of his ears. After five minutes of this "heavy petting" marathon, Bob called out, "Did you see that? When he's the very happiest he grins, closes his mouth, then sticks his little pink tongue out through his teeth."

Like the most attentive host, Buddy saw to my every emotional need, frequently interrupting Bob's and my conversation. He'd draw near to me, leaning in closer than two teenagers at a drive-in movie, and would lock onto my eyes from time to time, giving me the kind of eye contact that only means one thing: I love you.

At one point, Buddy suddenly surged out of my lap and dove headfirst toward my mouth just like his blueblood terrier days of chasing vermin down their holes. While this action may seem repulsive to nonpet lovers, it's a badge of honor for a Bond zealot like me to warm up a pet so much that he wants to kiss me on the mouth. I glanced over at Bob, who was wearing a big grin like the proud parent he was, obviously enjoying the way his little brother and best friend bonded so quickly.

This was so different from the Bob I remembered from our tense family gatherings. I had never seen this side of Bob before—so relaxed, and receiving so much personal joy out of not just seeing the other's happiness, but just luxuriating in the other's presence. I think that part of the reason we were able to be with each other in this new, more intimate way was because of Buddy. Animals have a way of creating a place of emotional safety in the room, a common ground of values where a different dimension of healing can begin. I've found that even among people who truly grate against me. If we are in the room with pets, or even talking about them together, we can instantly find something to share.

There's a woman in a nearby town who really would rather live some place else. Every conversation with her begins with a complaint about the very things about small town life that I value: that it's small, out of the way, simple, and unsophisticated. Many a conversation ends as quickly as it began, as I flee to the other side of the store so as not to be trapped in that negativity.

Then someone from her town told me that she lived with twelve cats and three handicapped dogs, a fact that overturned for me her reputation as cold and caustic. It takes a very generous and loving spirit as well as a lot of energy to care for so many animals. And she did more than care for them. The next time I saw her, I asked about her pets, and she warmed to me like the noonday summer sun.

Pet by pet, I asked her about the genesis of each pet's unique name, their nicknames, favorite places to be scratched, and what was the neatest and most unusual thing she knew about each of them. Pet lover to pet lover she was now unafraid to reveal her true self to me, a part usually reserved only for her pets. I not only didn't disdain her, I admired her compassion and appreciated the unique individual she was. All of that pain was relieved because of the connection to pets.

In a different way, the same thing was happening with Bob and Buddy and me.

While I honored his bright companion, admired Buddy's uniqueness and celebrated his little quirks, my brother and I drew closer together. Although I love his sons deeply, I'd never spent that much time in his presence praising them and agreeing about all their special characteristics, let alone touching them and letting them kiss me on the lips a couple of dozen times (as if they'd like to!). And you know, when your brother brags about his kids, the usual response is to dredge up something even nicer about your own. But Buddy created for us a place of total agreement where it was safe to be emotional, vulnerable, and honest. I realized that day was healing for us in many ways.

Sedentary Lifestyle—
A Heart-to-Heart Walk

AT THE TYLER STREET BAPTIST Church, the church my family and I used to attend when we lived in Twin Falls, Idaho, I wasn't the guy you'd go to for a Scripture citation or the one you'd pick to lead the choir. I was the official hugger. About a third of the way through the Sunday service, the minister would ask the congregation if we'd like to say hello to the people around us. That's when I'd seek out the ten or twelve little old ladies who needed a hug. Although I'd only hug them for a few seconds, in that instant I got a sense of what I was holding on to. A lot of these women had been widows for a long time and were starved for touch. Some of them gripped on pretty tight. But with others, I just felt that week by week, there was less and less of them there.

As a veterinarian, I'd developed a sense for which animals were going to make it and which ones were giving up. At church I got a strong sense that Ruth, a substantial woman in her seventies, was shrinking away, not in mass, but in spirit. When her husband died ten years earlier, that loss hadn't been too hard to take. They hadn't been close for a long time. But from the moment her beloved black Labrador retriever, Drake, died, she'd started to wither. "I'm next" is what she was saying, not with her lips, but with every fiber of her body. Her shoulders were beginning to slump and her mouth was frozen with loneliness.

I started taking Ruth out to breakfast from time to time to break her isolation. She'd wear her best dress and try to be a good conversationalist, but nothing seemed to boost her spirits. The day after one of our breakfasts, I flew to a business meeting in Houston. I was zoning out on the airport conveyor belt with my fellow harried travelers when my eyes grazed across an advertisement with an image of an elderly lady holding a dog. The caption read: "Like most people her age, she belongs in a home. Her own." Suddenly I saw Ruth's face superimposed on the lady in the photograph.

When I got back, I met Ruth for our regular breakfast, scheming away from the moment I extended the invitation.

"Why don't we go to the shelter and look at the pets?" I said cheerfully as I was paying the bill. But Ruth was on to me.

"Oh no," she said. "I'm too old for another pet."

"Let's just look for me," I replied.

In the car she was still resisting.

"I don't want to outlive the dog," Ruth declared.

I kept my mouth shut. I figured that if there was a love connection waiting to be made, I couldn't use logic. I'm all for people figuring out which pet best matches their lifestyle, abilities, and expectations. But I'm also for people falling in love with a pet for all the wrong reasons. No science, just soul.

Even though I'm a huge supporter of animal shelters, visiting there is hard on me. It upsets me that I can't take every one of the animals home. I walked behind Ruth to see which ones caught her eye. Also, I was purposely avoiding eye contact with the puppies and kittens clamoring against the cages, lest the Becker family find itself with an eleventh four-legged member.

Cage after cage, row after row, Ruth didn't even glance at the rambunctious youngsters. She eyed the graybeards: canines with white muzzles and jutting hipbones whose pace, hopes, and stage of life matched her own. About three-quarters of the way through the shelter, Ruth stopped suddenly in front of an old mixed-breed mutt a little smaller than a cocker spaniel, and stared directly into his eyes. The dog had been completely jet black in his youth, but age had turned his coat salt-and-pepper, starting at the now frosty tips of his huge upright ears.

The dog was too old to wriggle for her touch like the squirming litter of Lab-cross puppies pressed to the front of the next cage. He didn't get up, didn't lift his head off the floor, but stared steadily at Ruth. Slowly his tail started to wag. Ruth moved closer and the tail moved faster. She stuck her fingers through the mesh of the chain link door, and the dog studied them carefully. He rose to his feet deliberately and moved toward Ruth. He reached out his tongue and gave Ruth's fingers a gentle lick.

"If you were to take him home, what would you call him?" I asked, moving in for the close. But Ruth needed no convincing and wouldn't be pushed.

"I always come up with the perfect name for my pets," she said regally, unquestionably identifying the dog as her own. "I don't hurry it."

The next Sunday when I hugged her at church, she felt like someone had put in fresh batteries. I asked if she'd chosen a name for him.

"Oh yes," she said brightly. "Mickey."

"Mickey Mouse, because of his big ears?"

"No!" she answered, astonished. "Because from the first time I laid eyes on him, I felt like God slipped me a Mickey."

The Mickey that Ruth had been slipped is the health-inspiring relationship with an animal that can serve as a stimulus to exercise and engage with the world in a way that we, if left completely on our own, frequently decline to do. For years, Ruth's doctor had been lecturing her to get out and walk a little every day to try to manage her weight, keep her joints limber and her heart healthy, and to lift her spirits. But Ruth was easily winded and frankly, a bit depressed. Getting out of the house seemed like so much effort, and for what? But once Mickey entered her life, she *had* to get out to walk the dog.

When Ruth got out twice a day to walk her dog, the whole world of the neighborhood opened up to her. Mickey's pace was slow and steady, but he had an animal interest in sniffing out the territory. He took Ruth a lot farther than she'd ever have gotten on her own. Right away she dropped a few pounds and got more color in her cheeks and the light back in her eyes. People who had only seen her passing in her car on trips to the grocery or church now stopped to talk to her about her irresistibly cute dog. Those who made a big deal out of the dog by extension made a big deal out of Ruth.

As time progressed, Ruth developed quite a collection of dog accessories: brooches, earrings, scarves. She also developed pride and eventually optimism. Although it's hard to say which of these changes was most important in prolonging her life, she lived for five more years after she got Mickey. The week before we went to the shelter, I'd have sworn she wouldn't see the dawn of the New Year.

One of the amazing powers of pets is their ability to attack the chronic morbid condition of a sedentary lifestyle with joy instead of grinding discipline. One study found that pet owners were significantly more likely to report taking vigorous exercise three or more times per week than nonowners, and another study found that people adopting dogs sharply increased their walking time. Many studies of the activities of heart patients and pet-owning seniors report that those with animal companions get more exercise, particularly people with dogs. One study found that elderly dog owners spend on average 1.4 hours a day outside with their dogs. The kind of regular, moderate exercise you get by walking your dog fifteen minutes twice daily in the morning and at night exactly fulfills the U.S. Surgeon General's prescription for moderate, regular physical exercise. And you ignore that recommendation at huge peril to yourself and your family.

Most of us to greater or lesser degrees live our lives as Ruth had, trapped in cages of our own making. What paralyzes us deep inside is the toxicity of our high-tech, low-touch society. We see more people in the average day than we used to see in a lifetime—streams of people who pass briefly before us. Contact without connection. The goal of many days becomes "just get through, get home, shut down, hide out."

We speed through town, battered by the punishing commute, and flick the garage door open with a remote control. Entering from deep inside the bowels of the house, we trudge up the stairs, feeling like a human piñata. The neighbors don't see us, and we don't see them, thank God! We don't want anyone to interrupt us in our decompression chamber. Modern forces conspire to make it everyone's full-time job to sit with their fingers over the keyboard ordering everything—even our meals—off the Internet. The U.S. Centers for Disease Control statistics on our lack of activity are jaw-dropping.

Only 22 percent of us get the government-recommended amount of exercise. A compulsive few, about 12 percent, are the high-performance recreational athletes we see sweating it out on the Nike or Gatorade commercials. A quarter of us spend our free time implanted deep in the couch with no visible signs of movement except for the occasional flick of the remote. These 114 million Americans report no daily physical activity whatsoever. The rest of us—the great saggy middle—can be persuaded to take a walk or clean the house from time to time, but not very often. Unless we make a special effort to be physical, the culture supports our escalating sloth. We take the elevator, drive a block to go to the store or the drive-up window, ride our lawn mowers, and send an e-mail rather than walk down the hall and ask a coworker a question. "The continuing epidemic of obesity is a critical public health problem," said Dr. Jeffrey Koplan, director of the Centers for Disease Control and Prevention. "As a nation, we need to respond as vigorously to this epidemic as we do to an infectious disease epidemic."

The Centers for Disease Control and Prevention calls our physical inactivity the major underlying cause of dying before our time, more significant even than smoking. Approximately 250,000 premature deaths every year are caused by our sedentary lifestyles. A hundred years ago, the major causes of death were infectious diseases such as influenza, tuberculosis, and diarrhea. Once medical science tamed those, cancer and heart disease—illnesses directly related to lifestyle choices—leapt to the top of the list, with 55 percent of Americans dying of either heart disease or cancer. Since 1950, there's been a 37 percent increase in heart disease, the number one killer.

Diabetes afflicts as many as sixteen million Americans, with twenty-two hundred new patients diagnosed every day. Incidence of Type 2 diabetes is 60 percent higher since 1958. Teenagers are also suffering the unhealthy effects of too many hours before the screen. The most common kind of diabetes, Type 2, was once called adult onset diabetes. It was renamed to acknowledge the epidemic of it in children; now kids as young as six present diabetic symptoms that previously had been seen only in people older than 40. And it's a deadly killer. "Diabetes is already the number one cause of blindness in adults, amputations, and kidney failure, and it increases by two or three times the risk of heart attack and stroke," says Dr. Robert Sherwin of Yale University, who is past president of the American Diabetes Association.

Obesity—a major contributing factor in both heart disease and diabetes—is the true pandemic. The Centers for Disease Control and Prevention says obesity is up a startling 57 percent from 1991. Nearly 55 percent of the population is overweight, and almost 40 percent can be considered obese (meaning fat makes up more than a third of their body weight). About 5 percent of children were obese in the 1970s: today that figure is 11 percent. For all the public pronouncements about requiring our children to be more fit, our institutions don't support the idea. Enrollment in physical education classes has declined sharply in the last decade. In 1991, 42 percent of high school students took physical education classes, but that figure has dropped to 19 percent. The only state that requires students to take gym every day is Illinois. And many cash-strapped schools have sold mini-Pizza Hut and Taco Bell franchises in the school cafeteria.

The cycle of inactivity and obesity is linked deep in our animal selves. In his book *When Elephants Weep*, a brilliant examination of the emotional lives of animals, Jeffrey Moussaieff Masson discussed the German concept of *funktionslust*, the enjoyment of one's abilities. Masson described the lives of lions in cages in the zoo, who, despite having all the food they can eat and their medical needs taken care of, become depressed and listless. If an animal enjoys using his natural abilities, does he also experience frustration and misery when he does not use them? Masson asked. One thing is clear: when he's confined, he eats. Kris Berg, professor of health education at University of Nebraska at Omaha, said studies have shown that pent-up animals eat more food than their counterparts who roam free.

Many of us try, in our own fitful and well-intentioned fashion, to get off our duffs and get a little exercise. More than two-thirds of us say we want to take off some weight, or at least keep from gaining any. But the drop-off rate for self-improvement programs is steep. One study kept track of women for a year after they began an exercise program. Five percent decided to try a vigorous workout, and 34 percent pledged to stick to a more moderate pace. Within three months, 50 percent of those who chose vigorous exercise abandoned it, as did 30 percent of those whose goal was more modest.

Over the years, I've experienced my share of failed attempts to restore my youthful physique. In 1995, I'd entered my forties, and purposely quit wearing the kind of Levi's that showcased my waist measurement. "Relaxed fit" was more my style, along with coming to the last notch on a series of increasingly larger belts, and piling a few *X*'s in front of the *L* on my shirts. Like Bonners Ferry's version of Al Bundy, this high school quarterback was now a 226-pound weakling, in a body that felt like it was encased in slow-curing concrete. I didn't have to worry about peak performance in sports; I found simple tasks such as tying my shoes difficult. I not only couldn't see my shoes over the curve of my belly; I huffed and puffed as I tied laces I could barely reach. Slip-on shoes were catching my eye in Wal-Mart.

That year I gave myself—my imagined new self—a cherry wood-finished NordicTrack for a New Year's present. My new self was a better self by far. He required all the optional electronics to track his target heart rate, to model and time his workouts. I knew that *this time* it was going to be a cinch to follow the inspiration of the infomercial pitch people and their calorie-burning promises.

Seven years later, the NordicTrack is sitting in near-mint condition in the furnace room next to the rowing machine. Most of the homes I visit are a virtual museum of the past decade's other "gotta get 'em . . . they're hot" pieces of exercise equipment: Gut-Be-Gones, AB Rollers, Thighmasters, and Bowflexes. Exercise statuary, reminders of resolutions broken, patiently waiting for another January 1 or next summer's garage sale.

The problem with those fitness resolutions is that working out on machines is boring. When my prolapsed vertebrae gave me a middle-age mortality and mobility crisis, I reluctantly promised Teresa to take off weight by agreeing to thirty minutes a day on our home treadmill in the basement and an afternoon walk with our dog Sirloin. Huffing and puffing as my thunderous steps shook the treadmill, I felt like Bigfoot trapped on a giant hamster wheel, bloated and bored in the basement. I counted off the flashing red minutes on the display like they were marking off my death sentence. Not a single part of me focused on the joy of movement, the *funktionslust*. I'd find thoughts of business or other commitments flooding my mind, and awkwardly reach behind me to grab a pen and notepad to write them down.

The next day I was so sore, it felt like I'd just played a high school football game against a swarm of bulls. My body was so achy and stiff that I thought rigor mortis had set in. That morning, I skipped the torture on the "dreadmill," and by afternoon I had decided Sirloin could walk himself. But when I went past the front window, Sirloin's laser look said, "Hey, Dad, get off your duff and get out here." Helpless against those begging eyes, I did. I put down my work and picked up my gloves and snow boots.

Hearing every word, change in pitch, or squeak of the chair, knowing cues of your body language, even feeling your footsteps from the other side of your house, pets know when it's time to go for a walk and won't take no for an answer. Pets have lain quietly on the floor studying every twitch of your muscles, every movement of your brow. All my mother-in-law, Valdie, has to do is move her "lazy girl" recliner in some imperceptible-to-human-ears fashion and Shing-I, a Pekingese/shih tzu cross, springs to her feet in a martial arts move, rearing to hit the trail through the woods across the street from their house.

Those who study frequency of exercise report that even the most committed fitness buffs lapse from time to time. Once you start to fall off your goal, studies show, frustration and dissatisfaction grows, and what researchers call "self-efficacy" ebbs. Self-efficacy in exercise is the confidence that you are physically capable of beginning an exercise program and emotionally committed to sticking with it. The day after the new regime begins, efficacy is at its lowest. You're not feeling the wonderful effects of getting your body moving again, the grace of stretched and toned muscles and strength of weight-hardened bones. Determination can get you to continue for a time, but over the long haul, most people need a partner or visible, fast results to keep moving toward their goal.

People who exercise regularly have enhanced self-esteem, sleep better, report less anxiety, and experience mood elevation. But when the body is sore and you see exactly how out of shape you are, it's not much of a boost. Studies of what influences people to stick with an exercise program say that the largest factor is family support. Yet a dog doesn't just offer an encouraging word from time to time, as a well-meaning family member might. He knows when you're supposed to go, and he can make your life pretty miserable if you try to weasel out of it.

I've witnessed some hilarious attempts by people trying to fake their pet out of a walk, none of which ever work. People mouth the word "walk," spell it out, or write it out in the air with their finger, or pass each other notes. I had a friend who, when he wanted to skip walking the dog, would sneak out a side door, only to find the dog staring at him from a window with a look that said, "Nice try, buster!"

Janet Shulenberger, who with two employees runs Walking Four Paws, a pet-sitting and dog-walking business in Omaha, Nebraska, says that after briskly walking dogs for three hours a day, she often finds herself wanting to take a more leisurely stroll with her husband, Jason. But Russ, a bichon frise and miniature pinscher cross, and Ike, a toy poodle, take matters into their own mouths. When Janet clandestinely asks Jason, "Want to go for a *W*?", sometimes Russ will take Ike's leash in his mouth and drag him careening down the stairs to go outside. Or Ike will simply take the leash in his own mouth and stroll off, walking himself.

Just like a drill instructor at boot camp, Maggie gets her owner, Sid Goldberg, a former WWII Marine drill instructor, to move on command. He likes to take their walk around the grounds of their Sarasota, Florida, condominium at 5:00 P.M., but Maggie prefers an earlier stroll. Precisely at 4:30, this five-pound Yorkie bounds from the floor to the recliner with a military, in-your-face style, reminding Sid (as if he could forget) that "it's time." Sid can't fool her by pretending to nap. She paces impatiently beside his chair, sniffs at the leash, and finally stands on the arm of the recliner, eye to eye with her reluctant recruit. You'd think she was gearing him up for a ten-mile hike with backpacks. He gives up and gets moving.

More than just a nag to keep you on schedule, companionship is another factor that increases your chances of sticking to an exercise plan. A long-term study of people who adopted dogs found that acquiring an animal sharply increased the amount of time they spent out of doors. This particularly effects the elderly, who definitely need stimulation to keep moving. Keeping moving in one area keeps you limber and more confident of your capacity to get out and around generally. A year-long study of elderly people living outside institutions found that pet owners scored higher on all activities of daily living. Pets also make you feel safer walking new routes, with new neighbors, at odd hours.

With weight gain also comes depression, as it did for Maureen Keller after her fourteen-year marriage ended. She gained twenty pounds when things started to fall apart, about two years before the legal part began. Once they separated, she started drinking beer to get to sleep. By the time she moved in with her sister and her family in Littleton, Colorado, six months later, Maureen had put on another thirty.

Her sister Kathy and her family owned an eleven-year-old Lab named Bunker, who was moving pretty slowly himself. That year, the family had decided that Bunker was too old and weak to go on the summer camping trip, and they were going to have to board him. Every day, before Maureen began her efforts to find a job, she took Bunker on a long walk.

Kathy lived very near the Highline Canal, a canal that carries water from the Platte River and other sources into the nearby city of Denver. In the area where her sister lives, the canal meanders past horse and cattle ranches and serves as a watering hole for local wildlife. As Maureen and Bunker trudged along its banks, they saw snakes and foxes and dozens of different species of birds. "There was a big hill at the end, and we would huff and puff up that hill. We hated that," said Maureen of the early morning walks. "We would be exhausted, and when his family would come home at night, Bunker could barely lift his head to say hello."

Maureen also joined Weight Watchers, took antidepressants, and enrolled in a local gym. The combination really worked. She lost thirty pounds in three months, and soon thereafter got a job and was able to move out on her own. When she was packing up to leave, she begged her sister to let her take Bunker with her to her new home. Her sister refused, and Maureen agreed to move out only on the condition that the family continue to walk him. They did. Bunker has since been allowed to go on the family's summer camping trip. He's never missed a year. Maureen received one of her own dogs in the divorce, a beagle, who now walks forty-five minutes with Maureen when she comes home from work.

Recent studies show that even a tiny amount of exercise, as long as it's regular, can have a significant impact on your health. A recent Harvard study showed that women who walked at even a gentle pace—an amble, really—had half the risk of coronary artery disease of those who didn't move at all. A Finnish study demonstrated that those who lost as little as ten pounds reduced their risk of diabetes by 58 percent. As Health Education Professor Kris Berg says, "Walking your dog is hardly training for the marathon, but the health benefits can be significant."

A great side benefit of taking your dog for a walk is increased social interaction. A recent British study followed a woman with a yellow Labrador as she went about her daily routine for five days, and then five days without the dog. With the dog, she spoke with 156 people, or more than thirty people a day. Without the dog, she only interacted with fifty. Researcher June McNicholas, a professor of psychology at the University of Warwick, pointed to the interactions stimulated by the dog as the key to a better sense of psychological well-being. "This may help us understand why pet owners are frequently reported to be healthier than nonowners," McNicholas said. "Increased casual social contact can increase feelings of well-being and provide companionship."

The dog effect appeared to work, regardless of what the human looked like. In a second part of the experiment, they changed the dog walker's clothes from pressed trousers, a sport jacket, collar, and tie to jeans, scuffed work boots, and an old T-shirt and stained jacket. Oh, those British! In Bonners Ferry, Idaho, you'd positively stop in your tracks if you saw someone walking down Main Street in a sport jacket and tie. People passing by the British walker saw the dog before they saw the human's attire; social contact was significantly higher for dog walkers no matter what they wore.

You can see where I'm headed here. The National Institutes of Health estimates that Americans spent $33 billion a year on weight-loss products and services, when the best tool for our health is sitting curled up on our beds, aching to get us out in the world for a fraction of that cost. What your dog—in essence, a four-legged personal trainer that works for free—offers isn't some faddish wonder cure that will snap us back to our high school physique. He begs to break our cycle of isolation and inactivity, to get us out seeing the world again, walking and talking to our neighbors, and feeling more confident and content with our physical and animal selves.

Hippotherapy—Horse Sense

AS A THIRD-YEAR VETERINARY STUDENT, I dreaded the hands-on course on horses because I was scared to death of them. My father had been injured several times on horseback when he was a shepherd in the Jarbidge Mountains of northern Nevada, and he'd taught us to be very wary of horses. I knew the details of every time he'd been bitten, kicked, and tossed, particularly the vivid story of the time he landed on the saddle horn, wounding a very tender place. We had a horse on the farm briefly, and the one and only time I tried to saddle him, he twitched his tail and I dropped the saddle and ran.

I entered veterinary school never having ridden a horse, picked up a horse's foot to check its hoof, or felt the softness of its muzzle. In vet school, the three-month "equine rotation" would force me to spend up to four hours of the school day as a horse doctor in training—a glorified horse nurse. I'd be required to take their TPR (temperature, pulse, respiration), give them injections, feed them medicine mixed into molasses, change their bandages, or salve their wounds, sometimes standing on a stepladder to reach incisions on top of their necks. Yes, I would even have to go into their stalls alone.

The first day of the rotation found me, stethoscope in hand, in the dimly lit hallway of the large animal wing of the veterinary teaching hospital at the Washington State University College of Veterinary Medicine. The big doors at the end of the long concrete alleyway flew open so another student could escort a magnificent, injured racehorse to a stall. Racehorses shy easily, and the new surroundings had him spooked. I plastered my back as hard as I could against the wall as he pranced my way, his eyes wild with fear-driven energy, his head whipping around with the natural explosiveness of horses at the starting gate. I prayed that some other student would have to tend to that horse.

Unanswered prayers, as it turned out. The next day I was assigned to help this twelve-hundred-pound animal awaken safely from postsurgery anesthesia and rise to its feet. School procedure was to assign two students—one at the tail and one at the head—to wait in the padded, darkened recovery room to monitor the horse and help him to his feet when he woke up. A horse hoisting his weight to standing is a coordinated action under normal circumstances, but this one would still be drunk from the drugs when he tried. He might stumble.

Forget about *his* safety—what about mine? All he had to do was strike out with those feet, and I'd be down for the count quicker than the fall guy at a fixed boxing match.

The only noise in the dark room was the horse's deep, steady breathing, as another student and I tiptoed quietly to our places at opposite ends, so as not to startle him. The sound might have been soothing if I wasn't shaking so hard. I stared at his powerful legs, capped with hooves the size of salad plates. The contours of his muscles and veins looked velvety in the dim light. The minutes ticked by slowly, and he barely showed any signs of waking. I had a lot of time to think.

What was I really frightened of, I wondered? I had sailed through the small animal unit, the dogs and cats, and cattle and pigs (or food animals, as they called them), which I knew intimately from my boyhood. It had all been so easy that I fancied myself a leader of sorts. But I was no leader in the horse stall. I envied the calm of those who were confident with horses, and I didn't want to look like the klutz or scaredy-cat I was. I didn't want to show my weak side, my veterinary underbelly.

The horse was just lying there oblivious, while down at his hindquarters I was racing through fear, inadequacy, and arrogance, none of which would be useful in handling the horse. For this to go well, I'd need to wrest control of my emotions and keep the goal always in mind.

Horses are nature's own truth tellers; interacting with them forces whatever emotion you are feeling right to the surface. The size and power of the horse demands that you confront it. As renowned horse trainer Pat Parelli says: "Everyone who owns a horse is involved in hippotherapy."

Hippotherapy is therapy with horses, not hippos. *Hippos* is the Greek word for "horses," and hippotherapy simply means treatment with the help of a horse. Although people have been riding horses for therapeutic purposes for more than a century, the discipline got a huge boost from the courageous Liz Harwell. Harwell, whose legs were nearly paralyzed by polio, won the Silver Medal in dressage at the 1952 Helsinki Olympics, the first games where men and women competed as equals. Inspired by her victory over disability, a Norwegian physical therapist, Elsbeth Bodthker, established riding groups for disabled children that used the movement of horses to stimulate the muscle control and coordination of the rider.

Half a century later, there are hippotherapy programs in twenty-four countries, and the horse's functions have expanded to therapeutic riding for people with physical, psychological, cognitive, social, and behavioral problems, such as cerebral palsy, spina bifida, mental retardation, and depression. The North American Riding for the Handicapped Association distinguishes hippotherapy, which is horse-based physical therapy supervised by a licensed therapist, from therapeutic riding, which uses a variety of techniques to improve strength, muscle control, eye-hand coordination, and social skills. In both of these techniques, the horse serves as a tool to integrate body and spirit, whether the rider is an abused woman trying to find a positive metaphor for personal power, or a cerebral palsy sufferer working on posture and coordination.

Of all the animals with whom humans frequently share a bond, the horse is the only one substantially bigger: eight to fifteen times larger than the average person. Those who love horses continually face the issues of balance, power, and control. Even for those not addressing central problems like these, an encounter with a horse stimulates you. As I stood in the dark hospital room next to the slowly awakening horse, I had to face the consequences of my emotions. If I gave off fear, I increased the chances of a bad outcome. If out of arrogance, I tried to force him to do something, I put myself and my partner in physical danger. In order to get the horse to wake up without panic, I needed to find a way to get my body and my mind to reflect calmly and deliberately my intention to accomplish the goal.

Something must have clicked into place that afternoon, because the racehorse didn't even startle. Thanks to him, some great teachers and mentors, and the dozens of horses I've encountered in the last twenty-two years since graduation, I'm no longer frightened of horses. In my lifetime, horses have gone from foe to friend to family. We share our ranch with five quarter horses, and my family enjoys regular rides in the Idaho mountains for most of the year.

I doubt I'll ever be as good on horseback as Teresa and Mikkel, who can turn their heads slightly or shift almost imperceptibly in the saddle and get the horse to go exactly where they want, when they want, how they want. They have both gone beyond just riding, which, as Parelli jokes, is no more than the mere fact of not falling off. For them, a command starts in the head, goes through the heart, and is expressed through the limbs to the horse, thus exemplifying Parelli's description of the ideal relationship not as a servant and master, but as a partnership. In hippotherapy, as in the true spirit of any successful partnership, it must work both ways.

Riding a horse is what physical therapists call a three-dimensional movement. Each time you take a step, your pelvis tilts a little higher, a bit sideways and forward, then back. The horse replicates the sequence and the sensation of these movements for people with physical or neurological handicaps, reacquainting them with how their muscles are supposed to move. The pressure of the horse's hooves hitting the ground is another multidimensional movement that stimulates riders' knees, hips, and spines, far beyond what physical therapists can re-create with machines. The advantage of physical therapy on horseback, hippotherapists say, is that the movement is rhythmic without perfect repetition, constantly jostling and challenging the riders' balance.

"We believe the movement stimulates the brain, that it's a circuitry that goes both ways," said Joann Benjamin, a physical therapist and the medical advisor to the North American Riding for the Handicapped Association, which certifies approximately fifteen hundred hippotherapists nationwide. "We really like to feel that we are impacting the nervous system directly."

I've watched Joann Benjamin at work with kids with cerebral palsy and Down's syndrome, and adults with multiple sclerosis. In this kind of hippotherapy, the client doesn't really ride the horse because he's not controlling it. The rhythmic movement of a specially trained horse transfers motor coordination and balance to the rider, as a certified physical therapist walks alongside the horse, adjusting the rider's position and movements.

The therapy goal for Joann's client Dolly Dorsey is to post at the trot, which means to come up slightly and a little forward into a half-standing position in rhythm with the horse as they trot around the ring. To accomplish this, something Dolly did easily in competitive English riding before she got multiple sclerosis in 1982, Dolly must coordinate the movement of her solid, strong left leg with her substantially weaker right one. Through the horse, she also works on balance and strength training.

The therapy session at Ride On, a therapeutic riding center in Chatsworth, California, included forty minutes on horseback. Dolly used a walker to make her way from her car to Gem, a quarter horse whose small steps provide a controlled, steady gait. Joann had positioned Gem next to a ramp so that Dolly would be on a steady, wide platform next to the horse for easier mounting.

Three people attended to Dolly as she and Gem circled the ring or paused to work on specific movements under the shade of a tree: someone to lead the horse, someone to walk beside and ensure Dolly's safety, and Joann. The stewardship of the two people who handled Gem left Joann free to scrutinize and adjust Dolly's stretches and movements in order to bring her closer to her goal.

Once the session was over, Joann commented on how Dolly's strength and coordination had improved during the six months they had been working together. Dolly proudly positioned herself in her walker and walked confidently to the car. Even from one brief session, her right leg dragged less. In the four years Dolly has been going to weekly hippotherapy with Joann and other instructors as well as yoga classes, she's begun sitting up straighter, leaning less to the left.

At the age of sixty-six, Dolly isn't expecting complete recovery. She's simply happy that she's been able to hold off further degeneration.

Pat Parelli's seminars teach how to direct a horse not by force and intimidation, but by presence. Equal parts love, language, and leadership, as he likes to say. Pat is justly proud of the way the method forms a partnership between human and horse that enables people to get a horse to enter a trailer from fifty feet away with a simple voice command, or to ride one horse while instructing the horse next to him to vault an obstacle. Despite the international renown he's earned for his method, the work from which he's gotten the most personal satisfaction is with his son, Caton.

As an infant, Caton contracted hydrocephalus, an accumulation of fluid within the skull often called "water on the brain." The buildup of cerebrospinal fluid causes pressure on the brain and can affect vision, balance, and motor coordination. Caton's head began enlarging by up to half an inch a day. At three months, he slipped into a coma and the Parellis rushed him to Children's Hospital in Oakland, California, where doctors installed a shunt in Caton's brain to drain the fluid. After a few weeks in the hospital, the Parellis took Caton home to Colorado with a grim prognosis: if Caton lived, he would never walk or talk.

"Never" is a fighting word for Pat Parelli, a strapping six-foot, four-inch cowboy with a waxed handlebar mustache. "I just had this attitude: 'Oh yeah?' I'm going to figure out what it would take. What would it take? It just takes more love, more language, more leadership," Pat recalls.

The first challenge was Caton's poor motor coordination and weak lower limbs. From the age of six months, Pat had Caton in between him and the saddle horn as he rode around their ranch. Once Caton could sit upright, Pat strapped him on Sparky, his top horse. Sparky was so attuned to Pat's commands that he could say "whoa" from across the corral and Sparky would stop in his tracks. Parelli found this security to be an absolute necessity for Caton's next move toward autonomy. "Whenever you put a child on a horse, you're betting their life that this will work," Parelli says.

Pat watched Caton carefully on top of Sparky. He could see in Caton's face that he wanted the horse to move forward, but Sparky didn't get it. "His heart wanted the horse to go forward, but his body wasn't communicating the message," Pat said. "One day when he was ten, the lightbulb switched on. He got the idea he had to cause something to happen in his lower body to make the horse go."

As Caton understood this, he worked to make the lower half of his body reflect his intentions for the horse—a tightening of the legs around the barrel of the horse's body and a shift of the weight in the direction he intended them to travel. When Caton was able to do this with the horse, his whole body began to move differently. "His mind and body started working together," Parelli says. "He got the sense he could control his world."

After that lightbulb moment, Caton's horsemanship skills improved dramatically. "He went from being seatbelted in to being able to ride like the wind," Pat said. Prior to this breakthrough moment in the saddle, it took Caton ten minutes to walk two hundred feet because he dragged his feet and fell frequently. As he gained better control of his muscles, he could make that distance in a minute. Ten times faster. That's almost light speed.

Pat realized that it wasn't just his love, language, and leadership that was helping Caton progress. It was that the time on the horse was play. Pat is a serious and focused man underneath his genial cowboy exterior, but the horse taught him that he needed to be more playful.

"We all learn faster through play, through fun," says Pat. "What I discovered working with Caton was the key to getting him to achieve was through having fun."

In addition to the work on Sparky in the arena, Pat worked Caton out in a mental gymnasium. They'd do addition and subtraction with small candies. If he got the answer right, Pat would let Caton eat the candy. Pat would purposely transpose words. "Instead of saying, 'Go get the bag of dog food,' I'd tell him, 'Get the dog of bag food,' " Pat said. "Or I'd ask him to hand me the orange bowl when I was pointing to a beige cup. He'd look at me like I was dumb. I'd love it when he'd groan. When you get that, then you know you've got him engaged." As much as being more playful helped Caton, it also helped Pat become a better teacher.

As Caton's skill and confidence grew, he started letting Caton help round up cattle on the ranch, and eventually used him to demonstrate Pat's horsemanship techniques at horse shows and seminars. Caton recently graduated from high school, a pretty amazing achievement for someone who wasn't supposed to walk or talk. He happily participates in fund-raising rides for NAHRA, but he does not consider himself handicapped.

While Pat is not a trained hippotherapist, he understood the incredible power of the human bond to horses. "There are very few animals that when we get on them, we turn loose to their power," Pat says.

"With horses, we turn loose to their emotional and mental state. That was more support than any one person or doctor could give Caton alone."

Lisa Greer knew her son needed a different kind of support, too. She had been very concerned about her infant son, Nathaniel, from the day he was born. He was just a tiny little thing—she still calls him "a little peanut"—and wasn't gaining weight the way he should. At five and a half months, he weighed only eight pounds, and was having a lot of trouble keeping any food down. The pediatrician told her to relax and it would sort itself out as he matured. Nathaniel was just a small child with a delicate stomach and the doctor predicted the bouts of vomiting— as much as twenty times in a single day—would subside. They didn't subside, so Lisa persisted.

Lisa insisted Nathaniel see a gastric specialist. He placed radioactive material into his gastrointestinal tract, and radiographs revealed a congenital defect. Half his stomach was up in his chest just underneath the esophagus. The months of not eating properly had caused his stomach to atrophy, and the test revealed that it was twisted 180 degrees around, compromising the blood supply and raising the possibility of gangrene.

The specialist rushed Nathaniel into surgery to untangle and reposition the stomach. For a while, he seemed cured. But three weeks later, he was back in the hospital. Scar tissue from the first operation was obstructing his bowel. "The other shoe just kept on dropping," says Lisa of that difficult time.

In all, Nathaniel had three operations and six hospitalizations before he was a year and a half. Just when Lisa and her husband, David Blumberg, were beginning to lose hope, a pain management specialist at UCLA suggested nortriptyline, a drug commonly used as a tricyclic antidepressant for adults. It was a stroke of genius. Suddenly Nathaniel's nervous system settled and his stomach relaxed. Within a week of taking it, he sat up on his own and started to crawl.

After a traumatic two years in and out of hospitals, Nathaniel's condition was finally manageable.

Once Nathaniel's condition was under control, Lisa and David tried to help him learn all the things he'd missed because he was sick. He could crawl and pull himself up to a wobbly stand, but he couldn't walk. He was far behind in language development, although Lisa and David could tell by his bright eyes that he understood far more than he could express.

Lisa brought Nathaniel to Ride On for these problems, but her hope was that being around horses would help him in ways beyond stimulating his nervous system.

"He had so much adverse input from the pain and trauma from the surgery. I hoped that exposing him to the sights and sounds and textures of the stables would help desensitize him somewhat," Lisa said. Over and above that, she wanted to teach him some manners.

"Medically fragile, developmentally delayed kids come to be more overly reliant on adults," she said. "They can become bossy and tyrannical, with an imperious side to them, an outgrowth of being constantly tended to. I wanted him to develop a relationship with the animals. I wanted him to develop empathy."

At first, Nathaniel was having nothing of it. He buried his face and hands into Lisa's shoulder at the first session, and Joann had a hard time prying him off. Lisa was embarrassed, but Joann urged her to be patient. Joann quickly noticed that the one thing that caught Nathaniel's eye was the horses eating and pooping, two basic biological functions that he could not perform. Noting that, Joann got special permission from the management to allow Nathaniel to feed the horses carrots. He fed them weekly for three months, gradually getting more comfortable with them and the setting. Then he started mimicking them. The first piece of food that Nathaniel ever placed in his mouth was a filthy carrot from a horse's feedbag. "I was cringing at the thought of the number and kind of germs on that carrot," Lisa said. "But I was overcome by watching him voluntarily stick something in his mouth."

Five months after they started, Nathaniel was finally ready to mount the horse, his tiny head aswim in the smallest child-size helmet. His response on horseback was nothing short of miraculous. "More expressive language, more responsive to requests, and much more talkative," Lisa said.

In theory, the reason riding is so therapeutic to people with speech and language difficulties is again the unique way the horse stimulates the whole nervous system. "Speech therapy is a top-down profession," said Ruth Dismuke-Blakely, a New Mexico speech therapist who has treated her patients on horseback since 1981. "We work on the mouth and the brain, and don't connect it to the rest of the body. Speech and language depends on the integrity of all the other systems. The horse is a highly organized neurological system. A half-ton horse uses the tiniest twitch of a specific patch of skin to shoo away a horsefly. In therapy, it's like he lends his ordered system to a disordered one."

Nathaniel's speech therapist, Joann Schumacher, who lives only a few blocks from Ride On, decided to drop by and observe him riding. She was so impressed by his increased responsiveness, she decided she'd conduct his speech therapy sessions in the stables. Speech therapists increasingly engage their patients in real-life activities during their therapy sessions because they find the patient learns more quickly in that setting than if he or she is trying to reproduce random sounds. Hippotherapy fits right into the real-life therapy trend and, Dismuke-Blakely said, is approved by the American Speech and Hearing Association.

Nathaniel's therapist arrives an hour before his session with Joann, and she and he walk around the stables discussing the dogs, the cats and, of course, the poop. They pick oranges and admire the flowers. Once he is mounted, Joann Schumacher walks alongside, working on Nathaniel's speech while Joann Benjamin works on his body.

Lisa admits she's not convinced hippotherapy is the primary reason her son is learning how to talk at such a rapid rate, because, as she puts it, "The therapy world has descended on my little boy." She's cut back her work as a public defender to three days a week so she can supervise her son's various therapies, which include physical, occupational, and psychological, in addition to the work with the speech therapist and Joann at Ride On. Any one of these, or maybe the combination of all of them, is making a big difference for Nathaniel.

Nathaniel can't control a lot of the things other children his age have learned to master, such as what he eats and the movement of his bowels. He must remain stationary fifteen to sixteen hours a day while a tube in his stomach slowly drips nutritious fluid into his digestive system. Much of that is done while he sleeps, but Lisa admits he watches more television than she'd like, and spends a lot of time exploring the malls of Los Angeles in the stroller while he is fed. Lisa wants to give a sense of control over some things, while not allowing him to turn into a little dictator using tantrums to manipulate the adults.

"When he's five feet off the ground on horseback, adults are essential to his survival," she says. "He is the center of attention, but despite that, he doesn't always get his own way. They expect him to be polite when he asks for what he wants."

In addition to the physical stimulation of the horse, Lisa hopes to create for Nathaniel a sense of being responsible for his actions and attitude. The horse is just being the horse, walking fast or slow around the ring, depending on what Joann wants him to do. People bring their issues to the horse, no matter what they are, and see them reflected back in stark relief. "One thing horses provide kids is a risk experience that also requires cooperation," said Maureen Fredricksen, president of the Equine Assisted Mental Health Association, an organization whose members use horses as a tool in psychotherapy. Marilyn Sokoloff, a psychotherapist with a Ph.D. from the University of Florida, uses horses in her women's group therapy program, HorseMpower, for just this reason.

In traditional therapy, the patient and the therapist sit in chairs and discuss events that took place outside the room. In equine assisted therapy, the event takes place in the stall with the horse. The tactile nature of the therapy and the horse-to-human scale speeds things up dramatically, Marilyn has found. Having a live experience to interpret can break through logjams that have impeded progress for years.

For two years Marilyn and her partner, Memree Stuart, have held weekly two-hour group sessions in Memree's horse barn in Marion County, Florida. Marilyn makes a very slow introduction to the horse. In the first hour, as the women settle into chairs placed in a circle at the center of the barn, they hear the horses moving around in their stalls. As the session gets more emotional, the horses come to their stall doors to observe, enhancing the focus of the group.

The women must groom their horses for weeks before they are permitted to mount; at first, they only lie on top. "We encourage as much physical contact with the horses as possible," Marilyn said. "It's helping them to feel, period."

Exercising power and control are issues common to all her patients, who suffer from depression, anxiety, eating disorders, and many of whom have a history of abuse. "How could you be in control of this huge animal in a way other than beating him into submission?" they ask themselves. "How is it different than what I know?"

One of Marilyn's patients, Amy, had a history of sexual abuse. When she first started in HorseMpower in February, she had lost her job and was so depressed that her parents drove her to the sessions. Amy had been grooming her horse, Casino, for more than a month when she confessed to Marilyn that she didn't trust him. "Because of his size, the horse could choose to do whatever he wanted," Amy said.

Marilyn told Amy to imagine that Casino was the abusive person. Amy pushed tentatively, and Casino didn't budge. When Amy put her hands on the horse's chest, she pushed him across the stall, feeling a surge of power. At this point, the other women had gathered at the side of the stall and were cheering her on as she pushed Casino several times.

"She demonstrated physically where she wanted to put him in her life," said one of the onlookers. "No abuse, but she got him where she wanted him to go." The few minutes she spent moving the horse in the stall were a breakthrough for Amy. A month later, Amy felt well enough to go to a job interview. She got the job, and recently moved a thousand miles away to begin her new career.

"It's not power so much as being able to put myself first," Amy said about the effect of the horse on her relations with others. "I think that asking for what you want, speaking clearly to get it, and not taking no for an answer, is all about directing a horse and also about directing your life. What the program has done for me is to take me out of being an observer of my life and start me being a participant."

As I know from my excruciating minutes in the darkened room in vet school waiting for the racehorse to awaken, coming up against a horse brings your fears into sharp relief. The horse offers you a way to engage the root of that fear and a way to make progress. For people with physical handicaps, the horse lends its power from the ground up to stimulate and realign the nervous system. For those with issues with power and control, a horse allows the person to see the problem more clearly. Pat Parelli calls it love, language, and leadership; Marilyn So-koloff calls it balance, boundaries, and breathing; but both are describing the way the encounter brings up the struggle to integrate mind and body; to have our actions and our stance reflect our true intentions.

Animal Assisted Therapy—
The One-Eyed Wonder Drug and
Other Animal Healers

DR. WILLOW, A FOURTH-YEAR RESIDENT at the National Institutes of Health in Bethesda, Maryland, steps off the thirteenth floor
elevator at the Clinical Center and onto the pediatric oncology ward to
begin her weekly rounds. She is finely sculpted, with a distinctive tapered
nose and thick, mostly white hair, dark, dewy eyes, and yet she has no
boyfriend. Although she's smart, kind, and very intuitive, she's often
been called a bitch.

She parades by the nurse's station, where everyone on duty gives her
the eye. One nurse even pats her on the head. As she enters room 1301, Dr.
Willow is all business. She sits on the bed beside the patient, eighteen-year-
old Lucas Sparks, and then she is all ears. She listens calmly and without
interruption. Dr. Willow is good medicine, all right. It's evident from the
look on Lucas's face that he feels comforted by her presence, as if he'd just
taken a happy pill. Before she leaves to see the next patient down the
hall, Dr. Willow lays her head in Lucas's lap and waits for a hug.

Dr. Willow is a seven-year-old whippet who's been doing Animal

Assisted Therapy with her teammate, Linda Solano, of National Capital Therapy Dogs Inc. at NIH, for four years. They are one of more than fifty pet/people teams that come to the nation's premier publicly funded medical research center twice a week to soothe and rehabilitate patients undergoing clinical trials for very severe medical conditions.

The certified pet therapy teams arrive at a lounge just off the main entrance an hour before the therapy visits are scheduled to begin. All animals must be checked by a veterinarian for fleas, ticks, sores, or other skin conditions before they are allowed into the wards. Their human partners also must assure the doctor that the dog has had a bath within the last twenty-four hours.

Once the veterinarian has finished, a representative from the NIH's Recreational Therapy Department gives the teams their assignments. The doctors at NIH note if their patients, some of whom stay at the hospital for months at time, like animals, and if they would be receptive to a visit from an Animal Assisted Therapy (AAT) team. The animals can be used to boost the spirits of someone who is depressed, lessen anxiety, help with the management of chronic pain, or aid in physical therapy. A team might be called upon to provide a variety of therapies in a single day, depending on the individual needs of the patients on the ward to whom that team is assigned. Lucas, for example, has used Animal Assisted Therapy in every stage of his long battle with an obscure blood disease, leuckocyte adhesion disorder (LAD). LAD is an inherited disease in which the white blood cells cannot move out of the blood vessel to fight infection in the skin and tissue.

When he first arrived eighteen months ago, Lucas was depressed and withdrawn. What teenager wouldn't be? Plucked from high school to spend most of his junior year hundreds of miles away from his friends and hometown of Sparta, Tennessee, the twice-weekly AAT visits boosted his spirits. He'd just gotten a puppy before he left home, and spending time with a warm, friendly dog snug alongside him was a familiar security blanket, a little piece of home. After a week, he was communicating better with the staff. As treatments to cure his disease began, the role of his canine friends changed. He was in a lot of pain. Instead of simple, quiet contact, Lucas petted the dogs more. Studies of the benefits of our contact with animals show that petting a dog relaxes the body, lowers heart rate and blood pressure, and steadies breathing. Additionally, the focus on something outside yourself, away from your troubles and worries, is calming, too.

Lucas's immune system was compromised by the lack of good white blood cells, and it took him a long time to heal from even the most minor scrape. While they treated his blood chemistry, doctors also wanted to fix the sores that just wouldn't heal. He underwent a series of skin grafts for the sores on his legs. To get the skin grafts to take, Lucas needed to get circulation through his wounds.

Animals helped him here, too. The night I visited NIH, Lucas was a most enthusiastic dog walker. He was doing laps around the pediatrics ward with Willow at his side. I went to a different floor to observe another team, and later saw Lucas sprinting down the hallway with someone else's dog. Finally, when the visits were complete and the teams returned to the lounge where we met up, there was Lucas, trying to get someone to give him a dog to walk. Let him try to budge one of these dogs, I thought. While the human half of the team recounted what transpired in their sessions with the patients, the dogs were out cold, slumped against their human partners' feet. A couple of King Charles spaniels were asleep in a little red wagon that had been used to bring them in and out of NIH like a human-powered doggie motor home. One of them was even snoring. Anyone who thinks that Animal Assisted Therapy is a passive activity has never seen the animals after their work was over.

As the teams described how their patients interacted with the animal, Rene Stubbs, lead recreational therapist and nurse, took extensive notes that would later be added to the patients' chart. The teams gave candid opinions on whether or not they thought the session was effective, recommended if another visit would be helpful, and if so, what specifically they would do the next time the teams came to the hospital three days hence.

The seriousness with which Animal Assisted Therapy is conducted at NIH is a sign of its increasing acceptance as a therapy tool. While animals have been used to soothe the sick since the ninth century, it is only in the last twenty years that the medical community has started to incorporate encounters with them in treatment plans with people who have positive feelings about animals.

The Delta Society, which certifies the Pet Partners, draws a line between Animal Assisted Activities (AAA) and Animal Assisted Therapy (AAT). In AAA, a specially trained volunteer—a kindly middle-aged woman with a bunny in a basket, for example—might bring her pet into a school, nursing home, or Alzheimer's facility to get residents interacting and smiling. In contrast, AAT has specific therapeutic goals.

For example, AAA might have a volunteer bring her dog into the rooms at a hospital for a quick weekly visit with the patients who request it, while AAT might have a rehabilitation specialist using a specific animal/handler team for a prescribed amount of time to help manage pain. Another AAT physical therapy goal might be helping the patient work on range of motion with a new prosthetic arm by playing fetch in the hospital corridor.

To make these interactions successful, you must train both ends of the leash. To this end, the Delta Society established skill and behavior standards for AAT teams in 1990, and began certifying those who passed as Pet Partner teams. Last year found more than forty-five hundred Delta Pet Partner teams working in forty-five states and five countries, with a goal of increasing that number to six thousand teams by 2003. Delta has a waiting list of one hundred facilities who want to open their doors to Pet Partners, but there are not enough qualified teams to meet the demand.

Charlie Brugnola, a former canine unit police officer who quit after twenty-two years to train dogs, evaluates prospective AAT teams. His company in California's Apple Valley is called Good Dog, and he jokes that he takes the "pets from hell" and turns them into angels. His long experience with dogs has taught him to recognize an angel when he sees one, and that was certainly what he thought the first time he saw Sweetheart.

Sweetheart is a mutt, a happy, sweet stray who was set on fire by two teenagers in 1999 and left to burn alive. The brutes doused her with gasoline and used a long red BBQ type lighter to set her ablaze. A couple who was eating at a nearby fast-food joint saw the flames. They rushed out and wrapped Sweetheart in a jacket. Then they started trying to find a veterinarian who would treat her for free.

Sweetheart had third-degree burns over most of the lower half of her body. When they told Dr. Rick Mori how Sweetheart had been set ablaze, he had a hard time containing his outrage, but then he looked at Sweetheart. "She was wagging her tail and wouldn't cry out, even though we knew she was in extreme pain," Dr. Mori said. "She had a lot of feelings in her eyes, but the main one was, 'Let's give this a go.' "

Dr. Mori clipped away the charred hair and put her on IV fluids and powerful antibiotics to fight the inevitable infections that would threaten. He cleansed and bandaged her wounds with something extra to keep the skin moist. Then he offered a $1,000 reward for the capture of the two teens.

When word about Sweetheart got out, the community sprang into action. Her story was in the newspaper and on television and radio. People stopped by the clinic to contribute money for her rehabilitation; in the end, donations totaled $9,000 and the list of people wanting to adopt her nearly reached one hundred. Dr. Mori flew out a veterinary skin specialist from New York to do a skin graft on Sweetheart. They took six-by-three-inch strips of skin from the sides of Sweetheart's neck and ran these patches through a special machine. The machine macerated the skin so it was thinned to a larger piece of webbing that covered more of the burned territory. "Sweetheart had a chin tuck," joked Barbara Reyez.

Barbara is almost as responsible as Rick Mori for Sweetheart's survival. When she read the story in the paper, she dropped it and drove immediately to the clinic to ask if she could adopt her. When the staff told her about the list, she volunteered her services anyway. Barbara is an occupational therapist. She offered to come to the clinic with her twelve-year-old daughter, Lauren, to tend Sweetheart. So every day after work, for two months, Barbara and Lauren would sit with Sweetheart and comfort her as she took her afternoon whirlpool bath to stimulate the growth of new skin, thereafter rubbing moisturizing cream onto her.

Barbara's devotion to Sweetheart was in part to help heal her own wounds. Three years earlier, when she was vacationing in Mexico with Lauren, her lower half was burned in a propane tank explosion. Barbara was in a deep depression about her own burned body the day she had dashed to the veterinary hospital. She'd never gotten used to how the burns looked, and she was still in a lot of pain. She described herself as "sitting on the pity pot," and found that her prayers were in a rut. She kept asking God why this had happened. "If everything happens for a reason, please show me a sign what that reason might be," she said. When she saw Sweetheart in the paper, that was Barbara's "go" sign. Dr. Mori and his staff were so moved by Barbara's story and her consistent, compassionate care that they decided she could adopt Sweetheart.

Sweetheart came home resting on three velvet pillows: one at her head, one at her legs, and a tiny one to keep her tender legs from rubbing together. Barbara found that her time with Sweetheart worked better than antidepressants. When she massaged Sweetheart's legs, her own legs zinged with energy. "You can have a tragedy and come through," Barbara says of the lesson she learned from her dog. "Sweetheart doesn't hold grudges or feel sorry for herself."

Here's where Charlie Brugnola comes in. Barbara wanted Sweetheart to be a Pet Partner, figuring if she could have such a restorative effect on Barbara, it was her duty to spread this gift to others. She called Charlie, who was the only licensed evaluator in the area. He, too, had been horrified by Sweetheart's story, and had wondered what had happened to her. He was pleased to get a chance to meet this famous dog.

Charlie is not exaggerating when he says, "You've got to love Sweetheart." When you look her straight in the eye, her sweet gaze twinkling with hope and affection warms your heart instantly. If you step back for a longer view, you are shocked by her horrible disfigurement. She has a strip of hair down her spine from her tail to the midpoint where her full fur resumes. The burned skin has healed to a shiny, pale pink that is smooth and not tender to the touch. The only other sign of the trauma she endured is a slightly ragged left ear, tattered by the sparks from the fire.

Charlie took one look and fell in love. But for all her joy and affection, Sweetheart was unruly. She didn't know the basic obedience commands, a requirement for Pet Partner animals. But these were small obstacles as far as Charlie was concerned. He offered to train her for free. As someone with a decade of AAT experience with his German shepherd, Molly, he knew how powerful Sweetheart and Barbara could be in working with burn patients.

While he worked on basic obedience, he also worked on desensitizing Sweetheart to the unspeakable horrors she'd gone through. They walked the neighborhood where she'd been burned, and Charlie, using his cop training, asked everyone they met if they knew anything about the two boys; but it had been a long time and the trail was cold. At home, he massaged Sweetheart next to a roaring fire. As she got more comfortable with that, he'd occasionally flick a lighter near her head, which caused her to flinch and leave the room. His most clever desensitization was also the most eerie. He covered a red fire igniter with squeeze cheese and had her lick it off.

Sweetheart now works at the Arrowhead Hospital as a fully certified

Delta Pet Partner AAT dog. Charlie likes to take her to burn units, especially to people who are facing skin grafts. He recalled a recent encounter with an anxious and withdrawn young man who had stood too close to a bonfire and ignited his clothes, causing severe burns on his back.

Charlie told him Sweetheart's story and the boy explained his own, tearing up a few times as they talked. He reached out to pet her, and when his hand lingered on Sweetheart's shiny pink skin, Charlie explained that was where she'd had her skin graft. The young man looked at it critically for a while and said, "It's soft and warm. It doesn't look too bad."

They'd only been there for five minutes when the nurse came in to tell him they were ready for him in surgery. "He's getting reinforcement," Charlie said of the session. "Sweetheart abolished his fear of the unknown." As he was wheeled out, his last words were, "If that little dog can make it through this, so can I."

Being an evaluator means Charlie's also a talent scout. Different animals work with different people, so he welcomes a broad range of personalities. When a team passes the test, evaluators write a recommendation of which types of facilities are most appropriate for this team. If he'd approved a frisky border collie, he'd recommend the dog work at battered women's shelters. His high, light energy would chase away the blues, and the kids would love the breed's aptitude for tricks. An impassive cat he might recommend for duty with seniors. But one look at Lucky, Diane Francis's cosmetically challenged barn cat, would leave even the most tenacious AAT placement counselors scratching their heads.

Lucky is the runt of a late-in-life litter for Donna Francis's parents' sixteen-year-old barn cat. Born half the size of the others in the litter, he clung to life despite the fact that the left side of his face hadn't developed properly. He had only one eye, a cleft palate, and a crooked stub of a tail. Donna also feared he had brain damage because his walk was more of a drunken stumble. Donna convinced her parents to let her take him back to her apartment, where she raised him with an able assist from her toy poodle, who decided she was Lucky's foster mom and cuddled him regularly. After bottle feeding was done, Lucky gained weight rapidly, to the point where at fifteen pounds he outweighs all the other creatures in the house except Donna.

Despite his rowdy pirate looks, Lucky seems to believe he is the most beautiful and intelligent creature in the world. Ah, if we could all only have the self-assurance and aplomb of Lucky.

Lucky and Donna are Pet Partners. Donna takes him once a week to Fairview Elementary School in Sherman, Texas, where she teaches deaf children. An emotional glutton, he likes a lot of attention and will complain loudly until every one of the children has greeted him properly. When they are all seated at the table, he will take his place, which is right in the middle. He sprawls back and waits for the children to start petting him.

They love it when he decides they've had enough learning and spreads out on top of their schoolwork. He flops across their papers, tosses his head back, and looks up indignantly until all hands have reached out to stroke him. Lucky purrs so hard, he vibrates, which is great for these children. Before the kids knew the sign for purring, they would sign Lucky was "shaking."

Donna believes the lesson Lucky exemplifies for the children is that you can have confidence and high self-esteem, no matter what you look like. Not only does Lucky need their love, he's not shy about demanding it. "I think they see that Lucky is different but he is still doing very well. He's a very successful cat," Donna said.

Lucky also does AAT at the Reba McEntire Rehabilitation Center, where the message he delivers is quite different. People who are anxious and in pain are drawn to his easily heard purr and need for affection. Donna believes that the therapeutic value is how appreciative he is of what they can give to him. The patients are passive and confined, but Lucky needs them; they have the power to make him happy. But he's also a symbol.

People will drag their wheelchairs down the hall just to get a look at his unique facial characteristics. Donna remembers one woman who was upset that Lucky hadn't stopped by. She got out of bed and into her wheelchair and cruised around the rehab center until she found him. Once they were face-to-face, she took one long look at him and said, "My goodness . . . he's worse off than we are."

Two different populations regard the same therapy cat and come away with completely opposite messages. For the children, the Animal Assisted Activity message is: Life could be better. For the adults, the Animal Assisted Therapy message is: Life could be worse.

Not every animal has a healing effect on every person, so some programs offer lots of choice. Although dogs make up the majority of the Pet Partner teams (about 80 percent), all domesticated animals can be considered for the program. Currently there are dogs, cats, rabbits, horses, chickens, donkeys, llamas, birds, and pot-bellied pigs.

Volunteers at the Doylestown Hospital near Philadelphia work with the local Shriners Hospital on a regular basis as therapists there rehabilitate children with orthopedic problems. For example, for children trying to regain the use of their hands after major operations, Animal Assisted Therapy coordinator Kay F. Williams had her sister custom make a "busy-body"–type vest with snaps, little pockets with flaps and hidden toys, zippers, buttons, shoestrings, and Velcro to get the children used to manipulating their fingers again. The children enjoy dressing the animals up with scarves, ruffles, neckties, sunglasses. And laugh as they are doing it.

I've been describing scenes in which animals are stimuli for recuperation, and certainly that is a large component of their usefulness in a hospital setting. That, and as a release and relief from all the intrusions. The animals become, for the patients, something that subverts the schedule of the hospital and all the medical imperatives. During their session with the animal, time stands still and is governed by different rules. Not rules really so much as whims and fancies, a sneaked treat, a sly lick, the tactile escape of handling some soft fur and gazing into loving eyes.

In a time of trauma, a pet can also show patients, as pets did for the students who survived Columbine, that life will get better. The change of pace brought about by this brief encounter—usually no more than five minutes—can be so profoundly powerful that every single AAT human teammate I've talked to has seen their animal be the catalyst for someone who hasn't said a word in weeks or even months to begin to speak. Animals in the hospital setting can be just as important when it's a time for silence.

Cherilyn Frie has two therapy dogs, her Brittany spaniels, Belle and Teigh. Teigh is up and active. If a person needs a boost, Teigh knows just how to nudge, even to the point of placing his paws right up on someone's neck and demanding they perk up. But if Cherilyn is working at the hospice, she brings Belle, who is stoic and steady.

Frequently, the therapy session will start from the moment Belle and Cherilyn enter a room where someone is dying. Just the arrival of Belle allows the loved ones to release emotions they've been keeping inside. "For some reason, he gives them permission to grieve," Cherilyn said. "It brings them into reality, into the present moment, and they are able to cry, to speak, and to reminisce." Usually all the family members want a moment to hug Belle. Sometimes they take the hand of the person who is dying and guide it to Belle, particularly if that person had a pet in his life whom he really loved.

The most dramatic case of Belle's effect is Cherilyn's story of a close-knit Buddhist family who was holding a silent vigil in the mother's room, as they all knew her time was near. The family was especially distraught, as the woman was only in her fifties. Cherilyn asked if they'd like a visit with Belle, and the woman's daughter said yes, since her mother had had dogs all her life. Cherilyn was crouched down petting Belle as she talked with the extended family when suddenly Belle stood on her hind legs, sniffing and scenting as if she'd just heard a silent whistle. She lunged toward the bed and tried to climb in with the woman, responding to something that no one else could hear or see.

"I don't know what she's doing," Cherilyn told the family. "She's never done this before. I think your mom is very close to passing." The daughter burst into tears. The other family members started crying, too, and holding on to one another. They gathered around the woman's bed, holding her, and saying their good-byes. Cherilyn decided to take Belle out to the car. Her agitation wasn't helpful, she decided, and she believed the family needed some time to themselves.

Normally, after a two-hour shift, when Belle gets to the car she collapses in exhaustion. This time Cherilyn was having a really hard time controlling her. As they headed to her truck, Belle bolted and ran back to the glass entrance doors, trying to get back in. The doors opened when someone exited, and Belle took off down the hallway and dashed directly back to the dying woman's room.

It took all of her 110 pounds to control her thirty-five-pound dog, but Cherilyn wrangled Belle back into the truck. She returned to the hospice to write her sessions into the patient's charts ten minutes later, and found out that the woman had just died.

Cherilyn was conflicted about Belle's behavior. Her rash act had stimulated such an outburst from the family, but it wasn't directed at Belle. The dog had brought them into the moment and made them face what was happening as it took place, rather than standing there, as they had been, locked behind a wall of emotion.

Later, the daughter and young son sought Cherilyn out, and Cherilyn immediately started apologizing, saying that she hoped Belle hadn't done her mother a disservice. Instead, they had come to thank her. "It is a wonderful thing you are doing for the dying and for the family," the daughter said.

Modern medicine has the capacity to prolong dying, and often we face our passing not with the familiar faces of a trusted family doctor, surrounded by family, friends, and pets in our hometown, but in a foreign land: a high-tech urban hospital designed to prolong life. Pets, even a stranger's pets, have the ability to help ease our passing.

Cherilyn believes that the power animals have in these emotionally charged situations is that they speak the language of the soul. "They have innocence," she says. "They don't have reason and cognizant thought to cloud their perception. They are totally physically aware. They sense what is going on. They can smell it, and they can feel it."

When someone is very sick or dying, feeling emotion is the one thing many of us are too frightened to do. If we start to feel that flood of sadness and regret, how could we control it? In these situations, the animal becomes our role model for experiencing the overwhelming magnitude of what is transpiring, by being present, strong, and unafraid. The animals show us by example not how to control or suppress our emotions, but to experience them fully and let them go. Truly this is strong, life-affirming therapy.

Assistance Animals—I Get by with a Little Help from My Friend

TWICE A MONTH, CAROL KING gets together with her friends from the Poway Brush-Up Club in Oceanside, California, to put their assistance animals through their paces. The dogs play for half an hour or so, and then their human partners lead them through the agility course. They scale a small A-frame, run across a teeter-totter, and zip through the weave poles, exercises all designed to brush up their strength, stamina, and agility so they can better aid their disabled human companions. The toughest one for many of them is the six-foot ladder that lies flat on the ground. The dogs must step from rung to rung of the ladder, a delicate maneuver designed to mimic crossing a sewer grating.

When the dogs and their humans are spent from the exercises, they adjourn to a nearby Denny's for refreshments. One day a few years back, Carol and her assistance dog, Bubba, were being seated with the others, four in wheelchairs and several others with canes, when another customer started to object.

"That is not a guide dog and shouldn't be allowed in this restaurant," the customer insisted.

Granted, Bubba doesn't look like the stereotype of an assistance animal, nor does Carol fit the mold of what we traditionally think of as disabled. Bubba is not a supersized retriever; he's a seven-pound Yorkshire terrier so small that Carol frequently carries him in a cloth bag slung over her shoulder. He's not going to guide her away from a dangerous intersection or lead her safely up an escalator, but his presence is just as vital for Carol to lead a full and productive life. Carol has agoraphobia, and, prior to getting Bubba in 1996, she was too panic-stricken to leave her house alone and was on full disability. With Bubba at her side (or under her arm), she started leaving the house, accompanied by another adult. After a few months, she was able to travel with Bubba alone.

The restaurant manager tried to explain to the irate patron that Bubba really was a service dog, but the customer got more agitated, pounding the table and insisting that she call the police. The manager called the police, who asked for backup. By the time the four police officers arrived, the Poway Brush-Up Club had been served their meals, and their exhausted dogs were quietly sleeping underneath the table. Bubba was curled up with his best friend, Cooper, a bearded collie, nestled so deep inside the fur between his front and hind legs that he seemed to have disappeared.

The police asked Carol for proof that Bubba was a service dog. She produced the documents she always carries with her, because she is frequently challenged at restaurants and chain stores. She has copies of the federal, state, and local regulations governing access for the disabled and their animals, a card from the Americans With Disabilities Administration summarizing the law with an 800 hotline number, and a note from her doctor certifying that she has Bubba for a medical condition. After the cops reviewed her documents, Carol moved Cooper's hair out of the way to show them her sweetly sleeping security blanket.

The police then told the lady that Bubba was a legitimate service dog and left the club to finish their meals.

This nerve-wracking incident is a frequent occurrence for Carol and the millions of other Americans who suffer from invisible disabilities. An estimated 54 million Americans—20 percent of the population—are disabled, meaning they have or have survived a condition such as blindness, cerebral palsy, epilepsy, hearing loss, multiple sclerosis, Parkinson's disease, paralysis, seizures, or spinal cord injuries that substantially limits one or more activities of daily living.

This broad definition includes people who have survived cancer or have diabetes, as well as people horribly scarred by burns, or those who have other stigmatizing conditions, such as being too tall, too short, or overweight. The law also covers people like Carol with psychiatric disabilities such as panic attacks, posttraumatic stress disorder, manic-depression, and agoraphobia, among others. An assistance animal, as defined by the ADA, is any animal trained to mitigate a disability.

Carol's psychiatrist, Dr. Bryan Bruns, prescribed a small dog to help her with her anxiety and depression during that period when she wouldn't leave the house. "Some people can only leave home with children or their spouse," he said. "Bubba has become her safe zone, kind of like a security blanket. Once you face the fear and survive and face it again and survive, it starts to diminish to the point of no significance. That is what Bubba has done for Carol."

There are two components in treating depression: the biological and psychological components, says Dr. Bernard Vittone, president of the National Center for the Treatment of Phobia, Anxiety and Depression. Pets work on the patient's self-esteem and self-control, fight demoralization, and produce different and better habits. He's seen many successful cases where the combination of medication, therapy, and pets—a "pets and Prozac" approach—has turned depression into exuberance.

Agoraphobics frequently recruit a "safe person" who performs the same comforting function as Bubba does for Carol. The problem with a "safe person" is that people have jobs and their own lives, and it's very difficult for them to be consistently available. "With 'safe pets,' they are there constantly, and they're not begrudging or moaning under their breath," says Dr. Vittone.

New York psychologist Sue Shapiro, who has several patients who have assistance animals for their invisible disabilities, said for people with panic disorders, projecting their discomfort onto a pet makes them more comfortable. She compared it to giving a shy person a baby to hold and finding that it suddenly puts them at ease. With this "projective identification," they can focus on and speak about this discomfort, and be successful treating it, and by extension they are treating themselves.

Carol now travels the country speaking about Bubba and psychiatric service dogs. She serves on local commissions about access rights for the disabled, and has running feuds with several establishments that are less than compliant with the ADA regulations. "Is this a sign of recovery, or what?" she asks.

When most of us think of dogs that work with the disabled, we think of strapping Labradors or golden retriever guide dogs leading blind people safely through the streets. Our image of a service dog is so ingrained, said Ed Eames, president of the International Association of Assistance Dog Partners, that when hearing-impaired people show up to restaurants with their service animals, the staff frequently offers them Braille menus.

Yet only 3 percent of the country's disabled are blind, leaving a lot of room for some very unusual service animals providing unique services. For example, more than 10 million Americans suffer from an anxiety disorder marked by an intense fear of being scrutinized and humiliated by others. Social anxiety disorder (SAD) is the most common anxiety disorder, and the leading psychiatric problem after depression and alcoholism. Fortunately, these social phobias can be treated with drugs, psychotherapy, and pets.

If you are a manic-depressive like Joan Esnayra, you don't look different, even in a manic state. Joan, a Ph.D. geneticist at the National Academies (formerly the National Academy of Science), has suffered from depression all her life. Both her parents were mentally ill: her mother was bipolar and her father had posttraumatic stress disorder. Joan triumphed over a dark childhood that included sexual abuse by throwing herself into academics and sports. But from time to time, she'd be felled by depression. She went through a severe depression a few years ago, unable to leave her house and vacillating between deep depression, high mania, and rage. During this time she started searching for a Rhodesian ridgeback companion because she'd been very close to one during a particularly dark time in her childhood.

Sitting among a litter of eight ridgeback puppies, seven of whom were jumping up and scratching her face, Joan picked the one who simply curled up in her lap and went to sleep. She named him Wasabe, because her boyfriend had finally succeeded in getting her to overcome her disgust for raw fish and try sushi. Once she tried it, she loved it. In true bipolar fashion, she became obsessed with wasabe, the powerful, bright green condiment served with sushi. Wasabe earned his name because it's about trying something you're not quite sure of, and ending up loving it.

Over the next month and a half, Joan started to notice that when she was sitting at the computer for hours on end, Wasabe would head-butt her arm repeatedly with his nose. She would get frustrated at times and yell at him to stop. Then she noticed that the only time he did this was when she was fixating on the computer in a manic state. Wasabe was alerting her to the beginning of a manic episode. She understood the what, but why? She went on the Internet and started researching service dogs and found seizure alert dogs. If dogs can predict seizures, she thought, then Wasabe was in good company.

One problem with a psychiatric illness is that the disease attacks your ability to recognize your state of mind. If you have cancer or a broken leg, no one doubts you. But as bipolar people escalate into a manic state, they feel superior to the rest of the world, a dreary place they think of as way too stodgy and conservative. If you warn them of their change in behavior—the wild spending of money and days without regular food or sleep—they tell you that you are simply wrong. They are better off than you could possibly imagine.

"Mates are never believed. Doctors are often doubted. Whereas the messages of the pet are taken as bedrock truth," said Dr. Mark Smith, a psychopharmacologist and NIH researcher who specializes in mood disorders. "It's very hard to argue with the dog. Even in the worst of times, a basic logical function is preserved, and it's hard to accuse the dog of plotting against you. The dog is like a laser chop into their insight. I wish we could train more dogs to smell or sense this in its earliest stages."

Joan says the fact that Wasabe alerts to her manic states is the aspect that everyone wants to talk about, but it's only a small piece of how he keeps her functioning. She and Wasabe spend 90 percent of their time together, and his constant presence has helped her keep depression at bay and guided her back into the world. He even helps her when a random incident triggers bad memories of the past.

Recently she was flipping through the CDs in the Native American section at her local record store when she came across one by a man who had raped her in college. She froze as a crescendo of noise built around her, a sign of a panic attack. Her movements were robotic, as she walked up to the counter and told the sales associate what the man featured on the cover had done to her. She dropped to the floor and started talking to Wasabe. She kept saying, "This is the year 2001, this man can't hurt me now." She believes that if Wasabe hadn't been there, she would have probably ended up hospitalized.

Joan and Carol never know what will trigger a panic. The stimuli come without warning, and their defenses against them are inadequate. The service that assistance animals perform for those suffering from bodily seizures is similar, and just as powerful.

Sonya Worthy jokes that she is "young and decrepit." Although only twenty-seven years old, she's had her share of life-threatening experiences because of her severe juvenile onset diabetes, a condition that has made her legally blind. She lacks peripheral vision, and must go to school hooked up to an insulin pump. She also suffers from diabetic seizures. What allows her to be a full-time student at Southern Illinois University in Carbondale is Baby, a fourteen-pound rat terrier. Baby leads her down the streets safely, or sits in her backpack while she takes her classes. If she's biking or hiking with friends, Baby serves as a better blood sugar monitor than any she could buy.

When they walk to school, Baby serves as a guide dog, despite her small size. Baby stops at curbs and pushes her body weight up against Sonya's ankles to direct her around objects. "I wish Baby was bigger," Sonya said, "but she does a lot. She's saved my life more than once."

Four years ago at summer camp, when she had just gotten Baby, Sonya had a seizure in the middle of the night. Baby tracked down the cabin of the head resident and pushed and pushed at her until she woke up. Then Baby led her to come to Sonya's rescue. When they arrived at Sonya's bedside, Baby whined and cried to indicate distress until the doctor arrived.

If Sonya is about to go into a diabetic seizure when they are home, Baby stares at her, moves into her lap and places her nose next to Sonya's mouth, an indication Sonya needs to check her blood sugar level and adjust her food or medication. The hard work of Baby has reduced Sonya's seizures from once a week to one every six months. If she seizes, Baby runs to get other people or scratches at the door of the apartment to warn the neighbors. When she can't get help fast enough, she's trained to call 911 by pressing a big button on a specially equipped phone. Let's call it K911.

Baby was trained for these tasks by Marilyn Pona, a Branson, Missouri, trainer who runs Assistance Dogs for Living. She believes that almost any breed of dog can be trained for this work if the animal is close to the owner and the owner pays attention to the unique way the dog alerts them to their state. Marilyn starts training the dog by requiring the human to keep a journal so they can distinguish between normal activity and activity that she calls "communication behavior."

"Some dogs alert by leaving the room," Marilyn said. "Some start biting their feet. Some become agitated and aggressive."

The training is a long process and Marilyn spends a lot of hours with the human and the animal. When the human seizes, she gets the animal close to the human's mouth—even instructing it to lick the owner's lips—as she and others believe that what the animal is detecting, particular in diabetics, is a change in smell. When blood sugar is high, the diabetic emits a sweet, fruity smell and a sharp, ammonia odor when the sugar levels drop. "I've had a dog alert to a drop in blood sugar when the person was in the shower behind a closed bathroom door," Marilyn said.

Or in the beauty parlor. Bregda Neal's dog, Bubby, a one-hundred-forty-pound Labrador/rottweiler mix, goes with her to the beauty parlor in Ravenswood, West Virginia. He is trained to stay out in the reception area, about twenty feet away from the stylist, while Bregda has her appointment. One afternoon, after about fifteen minutes, he sensed something wasn't right with Bregda. He went to where her purse was stored, brought it to her, and placed it in her lap. Bregda checked her blood sugar level and found that it had dropped below the normal range. Bubby waited patiently while Bregda fished in her purse for some of the candies she carries for just such an occasion. Once she'd popped the candy in her mouth, Bubby resumed his place in the reception area.

Sharon Hermansen, a North Carolina trainer who worked with Bregda and Bubby, doesn't really like to think she trains the dogs. "I reinforce the ability they are born with," she says. She trained one dog, Boris, for Leigh Meyer, who wanted a way to keep her four little girls safe when she had epileptic seizures. In 1995, Leigh had been seizure-free for more than a year when she had one as she was exiting the freeway on her way to work, causing a five-car pileup. When the other drivers rushed to find out how Leigh was doing, they found her stiff as a board with her head thrust back, unconscious. By the time the paramedics came, she was conscious but she had no short-term memory, another seizure side effect.

"They were trying to get me to unlock the door or roll down the window, but I had no idea who they were," Leigh said.

In the aftermath of this terrifying accident, Leigh heard about seizure alert and seizure assist dogs. While her seizures are limited by medication, she still suffers them several times a year. At best, a well-trained dog could warn her before the onset of a seizure so she'd have a few moments to make sure her little girls were out of harm's way. At the minimum, one could be trained to keep her girls safe until the seizure passed.

Her search to find someone to train a dog for her was frustrating. A dog and training for it can cost from $10,000 to $20,000, far beyond her budget, and she'd have to leave her family for six to eight weeks of training. On top of that, they couldn't guarantee that the dog would alert. "One thing, if we fail, you'll just have a dog who really loves you," Marilyn Pona said, admitting that while her percentage is high, she cannot guarantee results. Leigh was at the local pet food store getting food for the family's two dogs when she saw a card for Sharon that said she specialized in basic obedience and training what she calls handicapped assist dogs. Leigh called immediately.

They chose Boris carefully from the litter. Leigh was attracted to a quiet dog who sat calmly in the corner of the room. Sharon recommended a more lively pup, one who was chewing at their shoes and seemed to catch everything that was going on. "You don't want the leader of the pack, not the alpha dog," Sharon said. "You want them to be protective but not too dominant or territorial. Say she had a seizure at the mall. That kind of dog wouldn't let the paramedics near her or her purse."

Boris was rambunctious. He ate clothes, socks, furniture, and remote controls. "Several times my husband wanted to strangle him," Leigh said. But Boris turned out to be one of the approximately 20 percent of dogs who are able to detect seizures.

That 20 percent number is not validated in a research study but it's the best guess of Mike Sapp, founder and straight-talking chief operating officer of Paws With a Cause, a Michigan organization that trains a variety of handicap assistance dogs. His organization has trained sixty-five seizure assistance dogs and twelve of those have alerted to seizures.

One day while Leigh was in the bathroom and her husband James was doing dishes in the kitchen, Boris started to whine and pace. James thought the three-month-old puppy wanted to go out or wanted to play, until he heard Leigh's head hit the bathroom floor. Leigh was having a seizure, which Boris knew before James or Leigh, even though she was behind the door in another room.

Boris was not very far into his training that first time he alerted. As he matured, he learned a lot of valuable skills to keep the children safe while Leigh had a seizure. She and Sharon trained Boris to keep the girls away from the stove. Leigh had once scalded herself when she seized in the shower and, as she fell, turned off the cold water. Boris knew how to turn off the shower and could pull the plug out of the bathtub to prevent the girls from drowning. As time went on, he grew more insistent when he sensed a seizure coming on. Leigh was working from home at the computer when Boris knocked her hands off the keyboard and scooted her chair across the room ten minutes before her seizure began.

"He would only get rowdy or annoying right before something was about to happen, a seizure or a really bad migraine," Leigh said. "He would do anything and everything he could to make me angry. He'd grab the remote and run off with it or do things he hadn't done since he was a puppy. Anything to get my attention." That was Leigh's cue to make sure the children were in a safe place and retire to her recliner so she could wait for the seizure to come and go.

Unfortunately, the Meyers' third daughter, Mackenzie, developed severe allergies to Boris, and they had to give him to another family. Leigh didn't think she would be lucky a second time around, but Lani, the standard poodle who succeeded Boris, turned out to have a much larger gift.

Lani sailed through basic obedience in three months and quickly mastered all the skills Boris had, except that she refused to stick her face in the tub. Yet Lani had other traits that Leigh began to appreciate. She stood at the front window watching the children if they were playing out in front of the house, and barked insistently if any of them strayed into the road. Lani did not like it when the littlest ones climbed on the barstools at the kitchen counter. If the family got separated at a department store—some kids with Leigh, and others with James—she'd be frantic. Her instincts told her to keep them all together. And when Leigh had a seizure, after Lani made sure the girls were safe, she sat on top of Leigh in the recliner, a paw wedged in deep at each side, holding Leigh steady to ensure she didn't hurt herself. Eventually she also learned to alert to Leigh's seizures.

Like Boris, her alert to seizures was to become a pest. She changed from her normally placid demeanor to a growling nuisance who tried to sit in Leigh's lap. Ten to twenty minutes after this behavior began, Leigh would have a seizure. So when one day Lani was whimpering and running between Darden, the Meyers' youngest, who at the time was six months old, and Leigh, Leigh decided she should check on Darden just in case. She got there in time to see her daughter have what they call a lightning seizure, a tiny flash of an episode that sweeps over a baby in just a few seconds. Immediately afterward, Darden let out a bloodcurdling scream, which Leigh took to mean she was suffering a migraine, just like Leigh does after her seizures.

Leigh rushed Darden to a pediatric neurologist, who admitted her to the hospital for observation. She hooked Darden up to an EKG to record her brain waves if she seized. Leigh and hence Lani came right along into the observation room. The neurologist watched as Lani exhibited the same fretful, whining behavior five to ten minutes before the EKG recorded Darden's seizures.

How are dogs picking this up? Do they smell something, notice a change in behavior, or something in the electromagnetic field? Most trainers disagree with the idea that the dogs are picking up on behavioral changes because so many of them are detecting a seizure through a closed door.

Deborah Dalziel, a researcher at the University of Florida, surveyed epileptics with dogs in a study financed by the Able Trust, a charitable organization devoted to getting jobs for the disabled. Ten percent of the dogs alerted to seizures. Of those, all 10 percent of the humans experienced the same five auras (changes in sensory perception, such as seeing white flashes or smelling things more acutely). So perhaps what the dogs are sensing is an electrochemical change brought on by the aura. Before a seizure occurs, there is increased electrical activity in the brain. French doctors reported in *The Lancet* that increased electrical charges in the brain are evident seven minutes before an epileptic fit occurs. One theory is that dogs sense those electrical charges much as they can detect a coming thunderstorm on a blue sky day.

"Often family members know when their relative is going to have a seizure. Mothers are the absolute best," says Dr. Bill Bell, director of the Comprehensive Epilepsy Center at Wake Forest University Baptist Medical Center in Winston-Salem, North Carolina. "Dogs may be like mothers; they don't know how they know. They just know."

Where does this canine sixth sense come from?

The predominant explanation points to a dog's extraordinary sense of smell. "Before a seizure, some abnormal activity is going on in the brain," says Dr. Steven Schachter, associate professor of neurology at Harvard Medical School and chair of Epilepsy Foundation of America's professional advisory board, in a *Reader's Digest* interview. "It's conceivable that this may result in sweating, or some kind of unusual secretion that a dog can perceive by smell."

Mike Lingenfelter's cardiologist, Dr. Eugene Henderson, suspects Dakota detects chemical changes in Mike's blood chemistry that begin to build up hours before Mike has a heart attack. Duane Pickel is still researching, with the help of scientists from the Smithsonian Institution, how his schnauzer George was able to sniff out melanomas. Certainly dogs who alert to the blood sugar changes that bring on diabetic seizures smell something awry because even humans, with our primitive olfactory equipment, notice those.

Perhaps, to echo Dr. Bill Bell's comment, the canine nose just knows. Dr. Larry Myers, of the Auburn University Veterinary College, has tested the olfactory capabilities of over three thousand dogs. His research has found that the relatively small human nose contains only 5 to 15 million aroma receptors, and has a correspondingly small portion of the brain dedicated to interpreting the signals those receptors transmit. In comparison, the dog has an estimated 250 million receptors. Besides having twenty to forty times more smell receptors than humans, dogs can detect certain odors with 10 million times more sensitivity than humans.

Dr. Jim Walker and his wife, Dianne Beidler Walker, are working to formalize the results Duane Pickel got with George. Jim compared the acuity of a nose to a high-end digital camera. To make a better digital camera, you don't need better receptors, he said, you just need more of them. Between our puny number of olfactory receptors and sniveling amount of gray matter devoted to smell, at best we humans can smell cheap cologne across the room, whereas a male dog can smell a bitch in heat across town.

There is an ancient contract between mankind and the dog, ignited around evolutionary campfires by physical touch, formed because of respect and mutual need. Man learned that wolves could be their eyes, ears, and nose, protecting them against lurking dangers and helping them with the hunt. Conversely, wolves, once they got a taste of earliest man's doggie bags, decided hunting was too much work, while begging was a surefire thing. Today, we rely on canines' extraordinary sense of smell to detect everything from bodies to bombs, drugs to missing people. When evidence and experience is taken in whole, the thought of a dog detecting cancer or alerting to epileptic or diabetic seizures doesn't seem all that remarkable.

Yet the dogs are more than just sensory mechanisms who graciously lend their superior skills for our health and well-being. Analogous to a mother knowing when a seizure is coming on, she is aware of her child's routine behavior and instantly knows what that subtle shift in pattern typically precedes. As Mike Lingenfelter and Dakota's veterinarian, Dr. Harold Krug, says: "I think a lot of dogs have a capability of alerting that you're having a heart attack, but a lot of dogs take a look at you and think you're not worth it."

Dr. Krug is joking, but he brings up a very interesting issue about these assistance animals. For the psychiatric service dogs, the Bond is everything. Most of the service they perform for their human companions is the security of a fail-safe presence they can lean upon during troubling times. Ask them and they'll tell you that like death and taxes, assistance animals are one of life's sure things.

Unlike psychiatric assistance or seizure assistance dogs, dogs for the blind are called upon to perform a number of impressive tasks. For this reason, Guide Dogs for the Blind, the oldest assistance dog organization, breeds them to a certainty of size and strength.

The day I visited Guide Dogs in San Rafael, California, the morning started at truly the happiest place on earth. I spent a precious hour with the puppy socializers, a crew of senior volunteers whose enviable job is to come to the campus once a week and play with the golden retriever, Labrador, and German shepherd puppies. The purpose is to make sure that, practically from the time they open their eyes, these puppies are used to friendly, loving humans.

The puppies have it pretty good right from the start. When they are born, their infancy is monitored by video cameras, which record how well their mother is taking care of them. Once they are weaned, they spend part of the day frolicking with their peers in a bright square of lawn that offers balls, chew toys, lengths of rope for tug-of-war, and inverted domed garbage can lids for them to flop around in. The socializers note if they startle easily, if they take the leash well, or if they are shy, and record their behavior on a permanent record.

When they are eight to ten weeks old, the puppies are transferred to puppy raisers: warm-hearted people who volunteer to tend the puppies for a year or more under very strict dietary, obedience, exercise, and socialization rules. The dogs go to work and out in the world with their family members, so they spend as much time as possible being an integral part of the world. The puppy raisers of each geographic area have monthly meetings, and representatives from Guide Dogs also make home visits to ensure that the dog is being raised up to standard, and to identify and resolve any problems.

At any moment, the dog can be dropped from the Guide Dog program or "career changed." If the dog bites anyone, exhibits a strong prey drive (i.e., can't stop chasing cats or cars), jumps at sharp noises, or can't follow basic obedience, it needs to find a different career.

Between the age of a year or a year and a half, the dogs come back to San Rafael for a full medical evaluation. They are radiographed for hip dysplasia, their eyes are checked for cataracts, and they are taken for several assessment walks by the training staff to see if they present any problems that make them physically unsuitable or temperamentally untrainable. Most of the dogs don't make it through the program; less than half of the dogs that come through Guide Dogs in any given year end up as actual guides or breeding stock.

When the dogs at Guide Dogs have been winnowed down to the precious few, the training staff takes over. They work the dogs every day, taking them to the shopping mall and familiarizing them with escalators, crowds, curbs, intersections, and the general chaos of urban and suburban life. Trainers career change even more dogs for behavior and temperament problems during this phase.

While these dogs are working their way through the system, classes of blind people arrive every two weeks to start training with their Guide Dog partners. The trainers spend the first part of the two-week session training the people to use the commands that the dogs have already learned. The trainers watch the students carefully because they are making a match of dog and human that is supposed to last eight to ten years. If the student is submissive, they can't pair him with a bold alpha dog, for example.

"The training isn't about tasks; it's about relationships," said Dr. Bonnie Bergin, president of the Assistance Dog Institute and founder of Canine Companions for Independence (CCI). "We need to match the personality of the dog and the person—interests and responses to things—

so that it's not an effort for the person to make the dog do what needs to be done. It's like a dancing partnership through life, a waltz rather than stepping on each other's toes."

After three days of training, it's "Dog Day," the day most of the students remember more than graduation. This is the day they meet their dogs, their new companions.

"You can't remember the meal you just had because we get the dogs right after lunch," said Ken Altenburger, a blind man who is the kennel manager at Guide Dogs. His dog, Honcho, slept at his feet while we spoke. "You don't eat lunch. You're thinking about the dog. You hear the dog's name for the first time, and it just starts sinking in right away. When we were introduced, Honcho wrapped himself around my feet and he never left."

The trainers start the teams off in the safe confines of the campus, mastering curbs and crossings. Immediately students start walking with a more confident stride and at a faster pace than they did with just a cane. After they are familiar with the commands and the feel of the dog, the trainers take them to the nearby mall and into San Francisco at night and during the day, so they can learn to feel comfortable negotiating a big city.

At the end of the two weeks, the teams graduate in a beautiful ceremony that gets you teared up even if you've seen it a dozen times. The puppy raisers bring their protégés up to the front of the stage and say a few words about how precious this dog was to them before they present the dog to the person who will benefit from this "transferable" Bond. Sometimes whole families come up to the microphone and each member, down to the smallest child, insists on praising the incredible love, spirit, and personality of the dog they will no longer call their own.

The most recent time I saw the ceremony, one family had written a poem and each member recited a line. In many cases the family presents a check to Guide Dogs to pay for the harness that will link their beloved friend to the new person in his or her life. Then the person who receives the dog gets a chance to thank the staff, the families, and the community at large for the incredible gift of this new creature.

The guide dogs are free to the blind people who take them, meaning that the organization does a lot of fund-raising to give these dogs to people in need. In some cases, civic groups such as the Lions or the Kiwanis regularly pay for a dog. In other cases, generous private donors sponsor one. It's an expensive proposition all the way around—it's estimated that each dog costs $70,000 to produce—particularly because of the staggering nearly 50 percent rejection rate. This is why Guide Dogs as well as other similar organizations such as CCI have intensive breeding programs that place strong emphasis on genetically engineering more and more perfect dogs.

The demands on Guide Dogs for the Blind and for the other disabilities, such as hearing loss, are great. They must be sturdy and fit, lean in weight with good hips, strong backs, and no visual impairments such as cataracts. To ensure this, the breeding programs for these organizations are intense mathematical strategy sessions where the breeding staff examines the genetic traits of a dog's ancestors five generations back to weigh whether or not he or she should become part of the breeding program.

The instructors in all of these fine organizations struggle to meet the changing needs of their clients. Guide Dogs was founded in 1942 to serve blind veterans returning from World War II. These veteran clients were mostly a physically fit population, with no problems other than blindness. Current students of CCI and Guide Dogs have other physical challenges, and many come from our increasingly aged population. "We're asking the dogs to be in some ways very gentle and calm and very manageable," said Patty Olsen, president of Guide Dogs. "But we're also asking them to work in a more complex environment, which might involve escalators and all sorts of various transportation modes. So that's a challenge." Another transportation challenge for the dogs is cars, which are getting quieter and quieter and more difficult for a guide dog to hear, therefore making it harder to read the traffic.

Unlike CCI or Guide Dogs, Paws With a Cause (PWAC), which trains a wide variety of assistance animals, has historically tried to take the majority of the animals it trains from shelters. Last year, 98 percent of the hearing dogs and 30 percent of the service dogs came from shelters, but it's getting harder to find dogs that make it through the program. In the first six months of 2001, only nine of the seventy-five shelter dogs made it through the six-month training program. The rest of the animals come from breeder donations, people donating dogs, or a small breeding program.

Up front, PWAC asks the client to videotape their home and be specific about their physical limitations and strengths, so they can match them up with the right dog for the job. After requiring them to come to the campus for two weeks of intensive training on subjects ranging from commands to dentistry, one of a team of over one hundred field instructors meets with the people and starts custom-training the dog and the person in their home, at work, or both.

Mike Sapp believes training the dog and the client in their home is superior to trying to serve the needs of a diverse group of disabled people in a single class conducted in a campus environment. "Compare the high-energy college student to the low-energy fifty-year-old mother," Mike said. "The same dog won't fit both people." The field instructors return to the home every eighteen months for recertification, because for most of their clients, particularly the older ones, disability is a moving target. "Their disability can change every year," Mike said. "If the person says, 'I used to be able to turn on the lights and now I can't,' we train the dog to do the new task."

PWAC trains dogs for many different kinds of disabilities. For cerebral palsy, muscular dystrophy, multiple sclerosis, and spinal cord injury patients, they train dogs to pull wheelchairs, open heavy doors, pick up dropped objects, turn lights off and on, get medicine, pick up the ringing telephone, put the laundry in and take it out, and retrieve food and beverages. Another unique training is for hearing assist dogs, who answer the door, get the phone, alert to the smoke detector by making physical contact with their human and leading them to the source of the sound.

Mike Sapp stresses how important it is to keep retraining these dogs and refreshing their skills. Eleven years ago, he matched Rosemary Douglas with a hearing assist black Labrador retriever named Ginger. He stayed in contact with Rosemary over the years, and scheduled retraining sessions to make sure Ginger was still in good shape as she got on in years. Recently there was a fire at the Douglas home, and Ginger escorted Rosemary to the door. When they opened the door, the rush of air blew both of them out of the house. Ginger thought Rosemary's husband would still be inside, as this was a time of day when he was typically home. Rosemary tried to grab Ginger to prevent her from rushing into the flames, but she couldn't. When the fire was out, the firefighters found Ginger dead of smoke inhalation. Her body was discovered right outside his bedroom door.

The most surprising condition for which PWAC and others, such as

Independence Dogs, Inc. in Chadds Ford, Pennsylvania, train dogs is Parkinson's disease, which produces rigid muscles and involuntary tremors. Parkinson's patients say the most frustrating part of their disease is feeling like a prisoner in their own bodies, rigid and uncoordinated. My father, Bob, had Parkinson's disease, so I was well aware of its potentially devastating effects. According to experts, drugs work well for tremors and muscle rigidity, but drugs don't work well for postural instability or freezing.

When a patient freezes, the brain is moving but his feet are not. He doesn't feel weak, so he keeps trying to go forward, but he can't. Freezing causes anxiety, and people tend to become socially isolated. Drugs seldom help for freezing, but dogs do. A specially trained assistance animal can touch the Parkinson's patient on the foot and he'll start moving again. It's like a laying on of paws, and the result is instantaneous.

Dr. Matthew Stern, director of the Parkinson's Disease and Movement Disorders Center in Philadelphia and professor of neurology at the University of Pennsylvania Health System, is a big fan of pairing patients with assistance dogs. Six years ago, at the urging of a progressive pharmaceutical company project manager who was looking for solutions beyond new high-tech wonder drugs, he was touring Independence Dogs, Inc. Dr. Stern suggested to founder and trainer Jean King that it would be great if she could teach dogs to tap a Parkinson's patient's foot when he or she froze. Jean said that was completely doable. After they were trained, the dogs could not only break a freeze with the tap of a paw, after a while they could anticipate the freeze before it took hold and stop it before it started.

Retired dentist Peter Morabito, sixty-one, from Potomac, Maryland, has had Parkinson's disease for sixteen years. He's had two assistance animals trained by Independence Dogs. His current dog is a two-year-old Great Dane named Niles. Danes make good dogs for Parkinson's because they are sweet, big, strong, and responsive.

Peter uses Niles for stability and balance, walking with him like a four-legged cane on his left side and using a crutch on his right side. Peter will sometimes fall forty to fifty times per day, and Niles helps him get up. Depending on whether or not the meds are working well, Peter will freeze ten to twenty times per day. Niles steps on his foot to break the freeze. The biggest benefit is that it makes him happy. With Parkinson's, in public people often thought he was drunk or on drugs. When people see Niles, their fear disappears and they're drawn to the dog, and by extension to him. "The dogs humanized Peter to the public," said his wife, Marilyn.

Dr. Stern was amazed at the emotional support the dogs offered these Parkinson's patients. "Pets can work wonders on emotional problems as well as physical ones," Dr. Stern said, noting he now regularly recommends pets for patients, not exactly something they taught him at Harvard or Duke Medical School. "The only problem with assistance animals for Parkinson's patients is it takes months and months to train them, and there simply aren't enough of them to meet the demand."

Perhaps the supply would equal the demand if there were more money in it. The disabled population is among the most poverty-stricken segment of our society. Many of them live on about $400 a month, which has to cover basics of food and shelter. For them, specially trained assistance dogs are prohibitively expensive, as is the cost of their upkeep. And despite their obvious benefits in making their human companions productive parts of society, insurance does not pay for them or help with funds for their routine and emergency care. "If something breaks on an electric wheelchair and you have to use the manual one, it's an inconvenience, but it's not life-threatening," said Tamara Whitehall, program coordinator for the Delta Society's National Service Dog Training Center. "If a service animal has a problem it must be fixed."

Ed Eames has a great story about Kirby, the dog whose problem he thought was unfixable.

Ed began to love his joyful second dog Kirby, who figured out where the bank was and which were Ed's favorite restaurants pretty quickly. He also was an adaptable traveling companion, a necessity for Ed and his wife, Toni, who is also blind. They travel the country together, speaking about disability and access issues. When he was six years old, Kirby was diagnosed with cancer in his left front leg, which hit Ed and Toni pretty hard. They felt very bad for Kirby, and really didn't want to have to get another dog for Ed so soon.

They happened to be lecturing at the vet school at UC Davis the day Kirby was diagnosed and shared the sad news that Kirby would need to have his leg amputated and would no longer be eligible to be a service dog. The students objected. The hall was abuzz with examples of other three-legged dogs who were still working, one of whom was a sheep herder. They insisted Kirby could still do his job if they worked with him to build strength in his other limbs.

On their way home, the Eames were amused by the students' optimism. A three-legged dog would be like a three-legged table, not very steady. Kirby would probably fall off the curb, they guessed. But after the amputation, Kirby was still game. He still got excited every time the Eames put the guide dog harness on Toni's dog, Ivy, and he still seemed very strong. The Eames decided to give it a try. They hired a neighborhood kid to build his strength with daily runs in the park.

"He had a very hoppy gait, but we didn't realize how strong he was," Ed said. When they were trying to get their dogs to jump in the back of a pickup truck, they moved first to help Kirby, but he jumped right in. It was Ivy, who was eleven years old, who really needed the help. The Eames reinforced Kirby's harness so the weight rested more heavily on his remaining legs, and he retained his job.

For a while, the Eames were worried about how the public would react. Would they think they were abusing this poor disabled dog? A factor in his public acceptance was his gay tail, one that curved around in a complete circle and was always wagging. Kirby was still so joyful and still loved his work. As time went on, they understood that he was important for more than just his happy attitude. He became a symbol and a frequent point in their lectures, representing what everyone in the disability community wants: the right to keep on working. As Ed puts it: "For a lot of us who are deaf and blind, the request is, 'Give us a chance. With a little accommodation, we can do it.'"

Seniors—Everyday Miracles
from the Love of a Pet

MY MOTHER, VIRGINIA, JOKES THAT when she entered her seventh decade, she changed her middle name from Louise to "Used To." As in: Virginia Used To be five feet, four inches. Virginia Used To have 20-20 vision. And Virginia Used To be a farm wife. It's typical that my mom would handle life's toughest parts with humor. People in Twin Falls, where she moved after my father died in 1996, affectionately call her "Crazy Virginia" because she roams the town armed with the latest jokes off the Internet and with a purse stuffed with cartoons (mostly risqué) to hand to anyone who stops to chat. "People always know they're gonna have a smile when they see me coming," she boasts.

You have to know my mom really well to spot the sadness underneath her perpetual smile. If you pull back a step from the cleverness of her "Used To" joke, you can see that her three punch lines neatly describe the landscape of loss as we age—losing height, sharpness of senses, and no longer performing the jobs that gave us our identities. The problem with the joke for me is that I still see my mother as she used to be. I don't think about what she's lost as much as about what endures. So what if she no longer has 20-20 vision. She's still got the sharpest eyes in the room. I can't see her shrinking because, to me, she still has huge stature.

My earliest memory is of her profile against the spring sun as she drove the tractor over the fields. This was a close-up view, not from the perspective of a child looking out the window at mom and machine on the horizon. I was looking up at her from a wooden crate my father had wired to the side of the tractor and my mom had padded with old blankets. By the year I was too big for the crate, I was doing chores. The day began at 5:30 when my mother entered the room I shared with Bobby, a glass of water in her hand, as she sang her version of reveille: "It's time to get up. It's time to get up. It's time to get up in the morning." And get up we did, because if we lingered in bed, she'd dump the glass of water on our heads, and we'd start the day sputtering.

By the time we finished our two hours of chores and milking the cows, my mom had a heaping farm breakfast on the table, a meal that provided more calories in one sitting than I now consume in an entire day. We always had bacon or sausage and eggs—poached, scrambled, or fried—hot cereal in the winter and cold in the summer along with pancakes, waffles, or biscuits. We drank whole milk from the Holstein cow that had tested with the highest percentage of butterfat in the herd. Despite the freshness and richness of the milk, it always tasted a little burnt from my mother's countertop pasteurization, which she performed with a device she'd bought from Sears as a newlywed. In addition to running the household, she was the bookkeeper, negotiated all the contracts, and managed the migrant laborers.

I saw my parents astride that land like two giants: my dad the colossus of the fields, bending nature to his will, and my mom managing our home with her wily negotiations. But as they aged, their sense of scale in relation to their surroundings changed. They went from having a large family around them, through which they were connected to the life of the community, to living alone. My sisters scattered first, then my brother settled with his family a hundred and thirty miles away. With a partner, I opened a veterinary practice only thirty miles away in Twin Falls, Idaho. Teresa and I started our family there, but we now live over six hundred miles away at the polar opposite end of the state in the Idaho panhandle.

When my dad retired in 1982, he leased the land around the house to another farmer, fortunately someone with standards as high as his. If he'd had to live on his land surrounded by someone else's shoddy work ethic, it would have shaved years off his life. As the years passed, I became very concerned about how poorly my parents were adjusting to retirement. Here they were living against the backdrop of their life's labors with only a few cows to look after. With no distractions and few responsibilities, Dad's mood swings were dramatic, and he was even more punishing to my mom. He was seeing a doctor about it and was on medications, but most days he just didn't know how to occupy his time. Sometimes he'd show up at my clinic and ask if he could sweep the parking lot just to be useful. I hoped if I got my dad a dog, it would help his depression. At a time in his life when fewer and fewer creatures depended on him, maybe a dog could be the one thing that needed him to get out of bed every day.

One morning I sat for more than an hour in the middle of a litter of miniature schnauzers trying to figure which personality would make the ideal pet for him. My dad had never had a dog of his own, so trying to decide which personality would mesh with his turned out to be harder than I thought. I chose the biggest, darkest male, one who looked like a gruff old fart, just like my dad. When I opened my coat in the doorway of my parents' house to reveal the wriggling treasure inside, it was love at first sight. He named him Pepsi, after his favorite soft drink, and the two were inseparable. Soon my mother got a schnauzer of her own that she named Ginger.

It worked magnificently. Everywhere that Grandma and Grandpa went, the dogs were sure to go. As they pulled into the driveway of our house, the dogs would be up at the window of the car like prairie dogs on steroids. Before you could hear their sound, you could see their mouths moving. When Mom and Dad's conversation deteriorated into griping or sniping or the endless loop replaying of a litany of health problems, I could get them out of it in a snap by asking them about the dogs, whom they doted on more than they did their grandchildren. In the summer months, they traveled with frozen jugs of water for them to lie next to in the car. They'd drive me crazy when I was a passenger, circling the parking lot for fifteen minutes looking for a spot in the shade so the dogs wouldn't be uncomfortable while we were in the mall. They always insisted on three levels of safety and comfort for the dogs: shade, personal ice packs, and the windows open or the car running with the air-conditioning left on.

At the beginning of life, pets teach a child responsibility and nurturance. At the end of life, they provide a way to hold on to those same skills. The senior fussing shamelessly over a pet is a sweet cliché of popular culture, the subject of countless cartoons. Seniors take such incredible delight at the things that they can do for their pets and the Bond between the elderly and their animals can get awfully syrupy, as anyone compelled to examine a roll of twenty-four nearly identical pictures of the many faces of Pepsi and Ginger would agree. Sickeningly sweet, yes, but also life-enhancing and life-sustaining, as medical and veterinary research increasingly demonstrates in studies of seniors and their pets.

Seniors who have pets have far fewer doctor visits than those who don't, according to a study of nearly a thousand Medicare patients by the University of California at Los Angeles Public Health Prof. Judith Siegel. The *Journal of the Royal Society of Medicine* reinforced those findings independently in the United Kingdom. Their study found that only one month after acquiring a dog or a cat, seniors had 50 percent fewer minor medical problems, such as painful joints, hay fever, insomnia, constipation, anxiety, indigestion, colds and flu, general tiredness, palpitations or breathlessness, back pain, and headaches.

Seniors were asked in a University of Montana study to make multiple choices from a list of reasons why they got a pet. More than 70 percent said companionship, 52 percent said love and affection, and 36 percent wanted one for protection: needs that are particularly acute for seniors.

Equally important for their health is having something to keep them active and out in the world. In a Canadian study of more than a thousand seniors, University of Guelph Community Health Care Prof. Parminder Raina used the Activities of Daily Living scale to contrast the self-sufficiency of pet-owning seniors to that of those who did not. The ADL scale asks if the respondents can perform simple tasks, such as getting in and out of bed, eating, dressing, bathing, and toileting without assistance. Pet owners were more active on the ADL scale; over the course of the one-year study, their scores remained essentially steady, while the non-pet owners' scores declined. Dr. Raina began the study believing that this effect would be true only for dog owners, because dogs are more active and demanding generally than cats. She was surprised to find that the ADL scores were higher for both dog and cat owners. "It's somehow related to the sense of responsibility, the sense of caring," Dr. Raina said.

In 1996, Colorado researchers tied pet ownership directly to increased activity in seniors. Elderly owners walked much longer distances than non-dog owners and had significantly lower triglycerides. The notion that dog-owning seniors are more active was also supported by a 1993 study by University of California at Davis Veterinary Prof. Lynnette Hart, who followed seniors walking with their dogs and without through a mobile home park where they lived. She found that dog owners took twice as many walks as non-owners and reported significantly less dissatisfaction with their social, physical, and emotional states.

Lynnette also noted the kinds of conversations the dog-owning seniors had. With or without their dogs, they talked lovingly about their pets to others, using their nicknames and discussing their habits and needs. Passersby stopped them and always asked after the dog. Owning a dog was a positive identifying trait for them, no matter what else was going on in their lives. Virginia "Used To" proves this point as well. Mom manages to work into nearly every conversation the proud statement: "I'm known to be owned by schnauzers."

One of the most interesting observations Lynnette made during this study was subsidiary. She discovered that those who didn't own dogs only talked about the past, while those who had dogs talked about things in the present. I find this side observation the most affecting finding in the study. So many seniors believe that all the good things took place in the past. For many of them, the days flip by like so many pages on the calendar. Their animal brings them into the present, into the moment—and brings value to that moment, too. The studies of how petting an animal lowers heart rate, blood pressure, and lessens stress note this same phenomenon—the animal brings the stressed-out, hypertense individual of any age into the present and, through the animal, the person finds something worthy here and now.

Perhaps this is part of the reason that our elders become even more dependent on their pets for emotional support when times are tough. Judith Siegel's study, which found reduced doctor visits for seniors who shared their lives with animals, was designed to examine how pets helped seniors through stress. For those who did not have a pet, stressful life events, such as losing a spouse or a close friend, resulted in more doctor visits. The number of doctor visits for pet-owning seniors stayed steady despite the losses.

An intriguing study conducted in Kansas by Carolyn Keil attempted to measure how seniors get attached to their animals. How did they spend their time together when the human was feeling low? Carolyn correlated stress and loneliness scores to the subjects ranking their pets' best characteristics. The loneliest, most stressed-out seniors ranked their pets' ability to gaze calmly at them as very important. The better they thought their animal looked, the more attached they were, too.

What's missing from this study is touch. Logically we know if you've got a pet you're not just gazing at his or her beauty from afar and trying to make a little eye contact from across the room. You're stroking that soft fur as you're looking into those loving eyes. "Often the elderly feel unworthy of love and affection. 'I'm old, ugly, stick-thin; who'd want to hug me?' " said Dr. Timothy Tobolic, a practicing family physician in Michigan and a member of the American Academy of Family Practice. "Pets provide that consistently and abundantly."

Touch is something that we all need, but that seniors get less of than anyone. University of Texas Nursing Prof. Mara Baun, who has done significant research into elderly and pets in nursing homes, observed the awkward way adult children hug their parents. "When you get to the point of physical affection, it's like a whole lifetime of interaction with that person comes into play with all kinds of things in the background," she said. "But with the animal, none of that comes into play."

What studies can't quantify, however, is that this interaction with a pet is a real relationship with a creature who has a mind of its own. It's not all gazing and stroking and lowering your heart rate. It's also laughter, distraction, and disputes.

Veterinary medicine is a small fraternity/sorority. I first met Don and Sharon Dooley in 1990 on a cruise ship where veterinary management experts like Don and myself had gathered for a conference. As a veterinarian, you're used to looking beyond the obvious to the obscure, and every time I saw Sharon at one of these events, there was less and less clarity in her eyes (not in a physical sense but in an understanding way). She'd be looking at you, smiling, with her Aunt Bee hair piled in a bun on her head, but her large eyes seemed clouded like a steamy bathroom mirror. The last time I saw her at the Central Veterinary Conference in Kansas City in August of 1999, she was like an animatronic wax figure of the Sharon I once knew and still loved.

In 1982, Sharon had had ear surgery and started complaining of terrible, throbbing headaches. A year later, her memory started slipping. As the years passed, her forgetfulness worsened. She would start to vacuum the living room rug, stop abruptly, and go to the kitchen to wash some dishes, leaving the appliance on. When Don bought a new car and asked Sharon to wait at the dealership and follow him home in their old car, she left before he signed the papers.

"We live ten minutes away, but she didn't get home for four hours because she got lost," Don said.

Diagnostic tests confirmed that his wife of forty-nine years had brain damage affecting her memory and her analytical skills. When her condition required her to be placed in a residential care facility, Don selected one four blocks from their home in Los Gatos, California. Don was left with the big space formerly occupied by the woman he shared his life with for so long and her formerly stray cat, L. C., which stands for "Lucky Cat." Don visits Sharon every day. At home he and the cat "are working on our relationship."

The first argument was about who really owned Don's desk. After Sharon left, L. C. started sitting right in the center of the desk while Don tried to work. Once Don was away for most of the day and L. C. had gotten locked inside Don's office. Don came home to find that L. C. had pooped underneath the desk and carefully covered up the shameful episode with papers he'd moved from the top. Don kept him out of the office for a couple of weeks. "For a few days, he wouldn't be in the same room with me, but he got over it," Don said. When L. C. was allowed back, he'd learned to keep himself to a corner of the desk. He's also learned which corners of the yard are safe from Don's surprise squirt with the hose.

Researchers can't quantify what pets bring into a home with that spontaneous interaction. Don's voice is full of love mixed with resignation when he describes bringing stuffed animals on his daily visits to Sharon, who now has the sweet enthusiasm of a child at perpetual summer camp. When he talks about L. C., the tone changes to irritated amusement. "If L. C. were to die, I'd go right down to the shelter and get me another used cat, an old guy just like me," Don said. "I had a granddaughter here for a while, but cats are better. He never sasses me and doesn't talk back."

Don's relationship with L. C. forms a thread of love and humor through his life. Contrast that with what it feels like to go into the home of a senior who lives completely alone. The senior who leaves the radio on all day so there will be another voice in the house. The one that you call whose voice seems almost fearful when she answers the phone because she hasn't heard it in days. With losses and illnesses mounting around them, it's easy to spend most of the day feeling sorry for yourself. For a woman like my mom, who was the hub of a large family, if she didn't have something to care for, it would be a profound and punishing loss of identity.

After my dad died, my mom was afraid to stay on the farm by herself. She sold it and bought a new home in a modest subdivision in Twin Falls that feels claustrophobic to me, especially when you compare her view out her kitchen window to the one she had from the kitchen window on the farm. Growing up, when we finally got a phone, my mom put a twenty-foot cord on the headset and would talk standing at that window, which faced south toward the Nevada and the Jarbidge mountains where my father used to herd sheep as a young man. There were very few trees, so much space, and everywhere she looked were our animals.

Now when Mom looks out the kitchen window, she sees four neighbors' back fences, a tidy rock garden with a careful arrangement of plants, and cast-iron statues of owls and deer instead of the real thing. The loss of the view from the kitchen window of the farm pains me much more than it does my mom, who never mentions it. She loves her tidy, all-white house, constructed completely around her tastes. The little spark of spontaneity that animates this atmosphere is her new schnauzers, Peanut Butter and Shelby.

My mom is far from lonely. She tells me that the dogs sit on her lap at the computer when she plays solitaire or writes e-mail. I know they are right there when she's talking on the phone because she makes me say hello to them individually. She volunteers at the local hospital and has a regular route of people she visits on a weekly or daily basis. Knowing she's got roots in the community helps me feel better about the fact that we only see each other a few times a year. And I think it comforts me almost as much as it does Mom that she begins every day by greeting her little buddies, and that the dogs fall all over each other with delight when she comes home.

John Stevenson, president of Long Island's North Shore Animal League, experienced the same kind of guilt I do about my mom when he thought about his elderly aunt. "My aunt would always want me to come over on the weekends," he said. "All the elderly I knew needed something in their lives to keep them busy, keep them active. Rather than feeling sorry for themselves and causing their children to feel guilty, I thought we should match them up with an older pet." In 1993 his organization started the Senior to Senior program.

The program matched seniors with pets who had roughly the same ailments and same pace of life. Despite the obvious benefits of pets to seniors, only 30 percent of those living alone have a pet in their home. Knowing that some seniors hesitate to get a pet because they think it will cost too much or that they won't be able to maintain it well, the program offered members pickup and delivery for free veterinary care and once-a-month grooming. The response was overwhelming, and rapidly the expense of running it started to eat up a huge portion of the league's budget. They stopped recruiting new members two years ago, but the program still has nearly five hundred members, about half of whom are in weekly contact with Program Director Jonnie Coe. Through the pets, the program has become an ad hoc social service agency for the seniors.

The seniors call to ask if someone can help them put their air conditioner in the window because "the cat really can't live in this heat." Or they'll call and ask if someone can come over and change a lightbulb. One of the drivers, a saint among us, now mows several of the seniors' lawns. They are obsessive, Jonnie says, about keeping their pets' vaccinations up to date, even when they forget their own. "This is it for them," Jonnie said. "For a lot of them, the pet is their whole life."

"My daughter fills out my income tax. My neighbor calls me to remind me to take my pills. I just gave up my driver's license, but they can't take my dog away from me," said Kitty Buckwalter, codirector of the University of Iowa's Center on Aging, characterizing the state of mind of the elderly. "In a time of cumulative and unremitting loss, the pet is the one constant. They are an enormous source of solace and companionship."

Beyond simple companionship, the pet forces seniors to maintain a certain standard of living. Scottish education expert Dorothy Alster described an elderly woman who kept getting respiratory infections because she refused to turn up the heat in her home. She didn't think it was worth spending all that money on heating when she was the only one in the house. When she got a canary, she started to keep the house reasonably warm because she was told it was important for the health of the bird. Better self-maintenance is a side benefit of maintaining their home and following a routine for the health and safety of the pet. The question "Why bother?" rarely comes up.

You may think a pet is a poor substitute for the loving attention of family members. Or that it is sad that these seniors have invested so much of their emotional lives in their pets. Yes, it would be better if they were at the center of a family and a community that invited them out and made sure they were okay. But if they aren't, the pet becomes a life spark. My friend Dr. Lori Sweetwood, a therapist who conducts group therapy at nursing homes in New Jersey, put it beautifully. "The quality of life is perception as much as it is the facts. As much subjective as it is objective. If you perceive you are no longer loveable and no longer needed, then you aren't," Lori said. "If your belief system shifts and you must keep yourself as healthy as possible to take care of this other being, you are worth being loved, and your entire perception of the world is different."

The pet brings the world to seniors in deeper ways, as well. Harvard Zoology Prof. Edward O. Wilson's notion of biophilia suggests that the human brain is designed to pay selective attention to different species of both plants and animals. Being around various life-forms, Wilson believes, keeps your senses sharper and promotes a feeling of well-being. This may be why pet-owning seniors consistently rate their health as better than those who don't, regardless of their individual maladies. If you believe the biophilia hypothesis, as I do, contact with animals and plants and the rest of the natural world is a contributing factor in keeping us healthy. This was brought home to me in a real way by the simple act of my father-in-law, Jim Burkholder, moving his chair.

Jim worked all his life as the head of his own logging company. Sometimes he had forty men working under him. Sometimes it was just Jim. Alone, he'd typically be up in the mountains for a week at a stretch, sleeping in a homemade wooden camper on the back of a truck. One day right around his seventieth birthday, Mother Nature gave him the signal it was time to retire. He was carving up a tree he'd just felled when the chain saw kicked back and drove the blade deep into his left leg. Even though the cut went to the bone and shredded muscle fibers flowered from the gaping wound, it didn't look too bad to him, so Jim got some Band-Aids out of the first aid kit, slapped them on, and kept working. Then a tree limb crashed down from a hundred feet in the air and hit him right on top of the head. After staggering around the woods for a few minutes trying to remember who and where he was, he drove down off the mountain, walked in his front door, sat down in *his* chair at the kitchen table, and said to Valdie, his wife of fifty years, "I quit."

Jim has more quirks and habits than a schizophrenic junkie. For fifty years he's always worn a green cap, always has a pocketknife in his right pocket and a pair of nail trimmers in his left pocket, unplugs the coffee pot when he leaves the house, and sorts all of the money in his wallet by denomination. And he always sits at the west end of the dining table by the giant wooden fork and spoon on the wall looking into the bowels of their tiny, dark house. Even when holidays and visits by relatives brought out the extra table leaves, his place at the head of the table remained unchanged.

Imagine Teresa's and my surprise when we came into their house shortly after he retired to find Jim sitting on the east end of the table. At first we couldn't form sentences. "What are you doing over there?" Teresa and I asked incredulously. Jim pointed out the window into the garden where the birds were at the feeders and the squirrels were playing tag on the side of the tree off the deck. "The squirrels make me laugh," he said simply.

You'd never have to convince Jim he needed nature. He'd made his living from the natural world and spent most of his working hours out in it so he needed it, but appreciating it wasn't on the list. When he started spending most of his days indoors, he craved nature for the survival of his spirit. Not the sight of Valdie's decades-old coffee cup collection in the cupboard, the fifties-era dark wood paneling covering the walls of the conversation pit (that never gets used), or the sagging bookshelves filled with *National Geographic*s from the time when Idaho was probably still a territory. Now he sees flowers in bloom, the fish pond full of koi, and, if he rubbernecks, he can even get a glimpse of the cottonwood-studded banks of the peaceful Kootenai River that flows no more than an eighth of a mile from their house.

He gave up the power seat at the head of the table because he wanted more time to laugh and more stimuli for his senses. Most days find Jim with his bird book trying to identify the same species of bird for the twentieth time (he forgets) or watching with his binoculars a gaggle of geese snoozing on a sand bar in the middle of the river. Keeping the senses active and stimulated is front line on the battle to keep ourselves young in body and spirit.

Old age doesn't just spring upon us. It starts at birth, and is the sum of the way we've lived our lives and handled what's come our way. As the Baby Boom generation hits its senior years, those planning for the coming avalanche of oldsters would do well to examine the data that supports the notion of animal companionship as a boon to the health of the elderly just for the cost savings alone. The fastest-growing segment of the population in the United States is the elderly, who now number thirty-five million and comprise 13 percent of the population. That number is supposed to double in the next thirty years, meaning we will have 70 million people over the age of sixty-five by 2030. Those who make it to sixty-five can expect to live another eighteen years, and women who survive to eighty-five will generally live to see ninety-two, while men can live to be ninety-one. As a class, their median net worth has increased by 70 percent since the turn of the previous century.

They'll have more quantity of life, but what will be the quality? A lot of them will be doing daily battle with disease, mobility limitations, and loneliness. Eighty percent of them will have at least one chronic illness, and 50 percent will have two or more: 58 percent with arthritis, 48 percent with hypertension, 19 percent with cancer, 12 percent with diabetes, and 9 percent with strokes. Between 10 and 15 percent of seniors will suffer some form of mild dementia, and another 15 percent will be severely affected by it.

Illness or not, these Baby Boomers are an independent bunch and will fight hard to hold on to their autonomy. Mara Baun and Barbara McCabe, professors of nursing from the University of Texas and the University of Nebraska, make a compelling case that animals have a role in helping us, no matter which of our senses desert us. They suggest guide dogs and hearing dogs if the senior's sight and hearing begin to decay. Old folks begin to waste away, they say, partially because they lose their sense of taste and smell so food just doesn't seem that appetizing. Baun and McCabe believed that pets stimulate the regular preparation of meals, and also offer social contact at mealtimes.

Apparently, some pet-loving politicians trying to rein in soaring health care costs feel the same way. A law that was passed in California, which was sponsored by Assemblywoman Helen Thomson, requires condominiums and mobile home parks to allow tenants to keep at least one pet, subject to some restrictions. Backers of the bill said that people with pets live longer and recover more quickly from illness.

If you end up being one of the 4 percent of the elderly population in a rest home, your family should look for one that allows you to bring your animals with you, has them visit regularly, or has a few residing there. As Dr. Lori says, the two central issues of the elderly are loss and loss of control. "They've lost every thread of control down to when they can pee and when they can eat. They are angry, withdrawn, sullen, and pretty hopeless," she observed. But things perk up considerably when she brings her dog Shayna to visit her clients at nursing homes. "The immediate reaction to this pet being there is everyone lights up. For that hour, people with Alzheimer's remember things. Memories are one of the natural healers for people."

Mara Baun decided to test out the effect of animals on people being admitted to a nursing or rest home because relocation has been implicated in increased rates of death for the first three months following this change. Earlier research had shown that people in rest homes were happier when a dog was present. In another study, those with birds in their rooms had better attitudes toward fellow residents and staff and rated their psychological health higher. Baun and fellow researchers Jill Jessen and Frank Cardiello placed caged birds in the rooms of some new residents and not in the rooms of others. They hoped a bright little pair of birds would ameliorate depression, loneliness, and low morale. The cages could not be opened by the residents, and others came in to care for the birds when the seniors were out of the room.

Researchers observed that health care workers and support staff spent more time in these people's rooms when the birds were there. One participant gleefully reported that her doctor came into her room each morning and sang the bird a brief song. No surprise, then, that the birds had a strong positive effect on the residents' self-scored depression. Many of them were very upset when the experiment was over and the birds were taken away. Several doctors who had clients in the home wanted to prescribe birds because of the positive effect their presence had on the mood of their patients, Mara said.

Increasingly, rest homes are bringing animals to live among the elderly because they see what a boon they can be to an otherwise sterile environment. While certainly I support this trend, I do fear for the quality of life for these animals if the staff of the facility isn't supportive of the idea. It's very difficult for a dog to live twenty-four hours a day at a rest home where the residents may be making constant demands on him, giving him no rest. The animals need to have someone who is their human, who takes them home at night for a rest and makes sure that his nails are trimmed and he is groomed regularly. Otherwise what could be a great intervention in the monotony of nursing home life can become a disaster.

The revolutionary Eden Alternative nursing homes, founded by Bill Thomas, a Harvard-trained gerontologist and family physician, are centered around the biophilia hypothesis. Nursing homes are, Dr. Thomas says, the only place on earth that have only a single species—old people—living with no life-sustaining biodiversity. This was the case when he began working at the Chase Memorial Nursing Home in 1991. Over time he and his staff brought plants, animals, gardens, birds, and children into the facility to make it seem less like a warehouse for the dying and more like a real home.

The staff installed birds in cages on poles in the rooms of whichever residents wanted them. They also acquired dogs, cats, rabbits, and chickens. The interspecies drama of the cats trying to get a better look at the birds, or the dogs who would sleep snuggled up next to the cats, created a lot of positive interaction between the staff and the residents, boosting the spirits of all. Industry wide, the staff annual turnover for certified nurse's aides is 104 percent according to Thomas. At Chase, that rate dropped by 26 percent. Over two years, the number of prescription medicines taken daily by Chase residents dropped from 3.7 to 2.4, and there was a significant reduction in the use of psychotropic drugs to control agitation.

The Eden philosophy has spread rapidly since the conversion of that first home in 1992 to the point where there are more than two hundred Eden certified facilities around the country. The one I visited in Escondido, California, is the kind of place most of us, in concept, would hate to end up. Silverado Senior Assisted Living facility is a last-chance Alzheimer's home, a place where all the residents have been kicked out of other nursing homes because they were too hard for those staffs to handle.

I'll admit to a little flutter in my stomach as I approached Silverado, that Baby Boomer flutter of facing my worst fear: that I would end up in a rest home not knowing the day or the time and being unable to recognize many of those I hold dear. I had in my mind the stereotype of the rest home with the residents sitting numbly in lounge chairs around the common room, drugged into submission.

All that trepidation disappeared the minute I parked in front of the place, a well-maintained, single-level building perched on a hillside just north of San Diego and surrounded by gardens and children's play structures. The place was alive. I was greeted at the door by a frisky yellow Lab and off in the distance saw a cat zip across the hallway. The first sound I heard was the booming voices of seniors making a complete hash of "Let Me Call You Sweetheart." Between songs, the underlayer of sound was the voices of fifty songbirds in cages around the facility. A man came up the hallway with his windbreaker on and a bundle of bedding under his arm.

"I'm going home," he said to Program Director Pat Thompson. "I've had it with this place."

"You are? Well, we'd be very sorry to see you go," she responded. "And I'm sure your daughter would be very surprised when she comes to see you tonight and she finds that you've gone."

"Well, I'm going and you can't stop me," he said, pointing to another resident. "He's driving me. We're both going."

"Okay, all right. But you're not in a rush, are you? Could you sit a minute?" Pat said calmly. "I'd just like to call your daughter and make sure she's not planning to come tonight. So why don't you take a seat right here and I'll get her on the phone."

Pat pointed the man to a couch, placed his bundle at the side, and called over one of the facility's eight dogs. The dog laid his head on the man's knee and looked up at him. The man started to smile and began to pet the dog. I watched for a few minutes, waiting to see how long this interaction would last and if the man would still want to leave. He petted the dog for a while and then lost focus, his mind a hundred miles or maybe thirty years away. When he stopped petting, the dog nudged his hand and brought him back into the room. He smiled and started petting the dog again.

This small exchange is only a moment but it says a lot about how this facility handles the waves of agitation that come over their residents on a daily and sometimes hourly basis. Alzheimer's disorganizes the personality and disturbs the priorities of the senses. "There is an internal world that is pulling them away from the external world," said Dr. Enid Rockwell, a psychogerontologist and professor at the University of California at San Diego. "They have lost the ability to filter out or at least prioritize, very much like schizophrenia. They are picking up the way their clothes feel on their body more than the conversation, but they can't speak, so we have no way of knowing. The problem is finding a way to reach them. Even the most impaired and bed-ridden will reach out to an animal."

In a different place, the man might have been met with anger, frustration, and sarcasm that could escalate his agitation. "What do you think you're doing? No, you are not going to leave," a staff member might have said, yanking his bundle from his hand and reinforcing his feeling of powerlessness. At Silverado, he was gently delayed and distracted, and quickly he calmed down on his own.

"As their short-term memory and language skills decline, emotions and intuition heighten," said Pat. "For a long time when this disease begins, the person knows he is behaving inappropriately, but he can't stop himself. It leads to a lot of frustration and anger. Residents who see him in the hallway don't know if he's finding a thought or if he's absolutely bewildered and doesn't know what this place is. I can take that loss and save that moment. Put enough moments together, you make a day."

The effect this dog had on this man is supported by the studies of Alzheimer's patients and Animal Assisted Therapy visits in nursing homes. When animals are present, the Alzheimer's sufferers are more responsive generally and more positive. In a study by Baun, McCabe, Kathryn Batson, and Carol Wilson, the patients smiled, leaned forward, touched, and talked more. They also expressed more positive emotion and praise, such as saying, "You understand, don't you?" and "That's a nice dog. You're a good dog, aren't you?"

There is no definitive cause or cure for Alzheimer's, so treatment focuses on reducing some of the symptoms and modifying the environment to reduce agitation. One way to do this, Kitty Buckwalter observed in her study of social behavior and institutionalized Alzheimer's patients, is to make sure that the stimulation around them matches their level of functioning. Too much, and they become dangerously agitated. Too little, and they become isolated and withdrawn.

What Baun and McCabe found in their study of Alzheimer's patients and dogs is that a trained therapy animal in most cases perfectly matches the level of stimulation the Alzheimer's patient needs. It can also serve as a buffer in disputes between patients. In a Buckwalter study of Alzheimer's patients in a veteran's hospital, when residents started to argue, the dog would get in between them and start to bark. "As soon as they focused on the barking, they forgot what they were arguing about," Buckwalter said.

At Silverado, both elements are in play: the positive distracting ability of the pets and a positive atmosphere for the residents.

"We're not a 'no' community," said Kathy Greene, facility director. "When you are caring for someone in a home, their world is full of 'no': Don't touch that. Don't go out that door. Here we want to greet them with 'yes.' If they want to go out and water the tomato plants twenty times a day, so what? If the plants die, we have other residents who like to plant new ones."

Following the Eden philosophy, the staff consciously tries to give the residents as much autonomy as it is safe for them to handle. There are set mealtimes, but there is also a fifties-style diner attached to the dining room where residents can get a cup of coffee or a meal most of the day. The nurses' station in the center of the facility was replaced by a country kitchen where the refrigerator is available and there is ample food and supervised cooking projects for those who miss being able to make something for themselves. Some residents like to be useful and are pulled into service folding the laundry in the morning. Residents are free to rearrange the furniture in their room as often as they feel like it, with the help of the staff.

These simple choices have a profound effect on the well-being of the residents. One resident had been kicked out of her previous rest home because of her violent agitation every morning right around breakfast. She was unable to communicate that she'd been raised in a genteel home in the South and rarely had been up before 10:00 A.M. Getting her up at 8:00 A.M. for breakfast set her off on the wrong foot. When she came to Silverado and was able to get her morning coffee at the diner around 11:00 A.M., her agitation largely disappeared.

The company keeps records of their success in reaching this population, which many consider to be unreachable. Since January 1997, 175 people who came in wheelchairs started walking again, 107 who had been hand-fed by staff in other facilities regained the ability to feed themselves, thirty-seven became continent, along with a 46 percent reduction in psychotropic drugs.

Families frequently see the effectiveness of the animal therapy on their loved ones where scientific research hasn't made the connection just yet. Kitty Buckwalter notes that the families of the veterans at the hospital where she was conducting her research deemed the dog who worked there extremely important to their loved ones' well-being. When the hospital had a problem paying for the shots and veterinarian visits for the dog, the families established a fund for that purpose, which they all contributed to.

The elderly in Senior to Senior got from their pets the same thing Lynnette Hart's seniors walking their dogs in the trailer park did. The pet was a bridge from their homes to the world, a world that increasingly was rushing by faster and faster, leaving them farther and farther behind. With their pets as the access point, they greet the world as people who care and love, and receive both back.

PART TWO

The Pet Prescription

Finding the Best Pet for What Ails You

IF YOU BELIEVE PETS HELP make and keep people healthy, one nagging question might challenge that conviction: If more than 60 percent of American homes contain pets, why aren't most of us a lot healthier? For a prescription to work effectively, we must take it as directed. Most of us are not getting as much as we can out of the Bond. The stories in this book show that the people with the deepest Bonds with their pets get the greatest health benefits.

Although I have always lived surrounded by animals, I never really tapped into the healthful powers of my menagerie until I got sick. When illness forced me to shift my focus to the here and now, my pets became my physical therapists, pain management consultants, personal trainers, and psychological counselors. I only received these benefits because I took the time to enhance our Bond: to slow to their pace, follow their instincts, and begin, like them, to listen to my heart and express gratitude for simpler gifts.

This section offers a guide to building the Bond, a process that starts with selecting the perfect pet match for your lifestyle, expectations, and needs; there are even specific types of pets recommended for different medical conditions. I'll move from there to tips on pet socialization and training, including some proven tactics to get along better with the animals already in your home.

I'll also share with you what I learned along the way in deepening the Bond with my animals. I interviewed experts at top teaching hospitals and street-smart authorities, ranging from a senior *Cat Fancy* magazine editor to a hippie who specializes in feline bodywork on the break room counter at the local shelter. Surprisingly, the steps I took to enhance the Bond with my pets were easily incorporated into my everyday interactions with them. I could see that even if I was not ill and off life's merry-go-round, these steps would not be time drainers. Most important, a rewarding transformation took place before my very eyes! By optimizing my time with my pets, they became models of complete contentment, and by the end of the day I, too, felt revived and rejuvenated.

Choosing Your Pets Wisely— Selecting the Right Make and Model

In this section, we will explore how to select the characteristics in your pet that best suit your lifestyle and complement your personality. The first challenge in determining the best make and model of a pet that's right for you is what I call the Great Car-Pet Debate. Take a moment to consider how much time you invested in selecting your last car, compared to your last pet. I'm willing to bet that you spent more time picking out your version of a Range Rover than you did the right Rover, despite the fact that our pets outlast two or three cars. A new car buyer might study consumer guides, review color schemes, take test-drives, and include other family members in the decision. But when it comes to selecting a pet, we tend to act purely on emotions, seeking very little information. The phenomenon of love at first sight certainly rings true when we see an adorable puppy or kitten. Puppy or kitty love is a powerful force of nature, one I confess I'm not immune to.

I have pulled into the parking lot of Wal-Mart, the country's largest ad hoc chain of pet adoption centers, to see a huge sign leaning up against a cardboard box that says FREE PUPPIES! or FREE KITTENS! Although

I know better, I, too, have been sucked in by that invisible, irresistible retractor beam that summons harried shoppers—people who previously didn't have a minute to spare—to jostle *ooh*ing and *aah*ing through the crowd just to have a look.

The spring after we moved to Bonners Ferry, Teresa was driving as we headed to our favorite cove at the lake for a picnic. Scooter and I were riding double-barrel shotgun (she was on my lap in the passenger seat), and we stopped at a Saturday outdoor market to get some fresh baked bread. I turned from buying the bread to find Teresa and my daughter, Mikkel, thrusting two identical cream-colored furballs—eight-week-old Himalayan-mix kitties—right into my face. "Can we take them home?" they begged in stereo.

"Absolutely not," I replied responsibly. "We don't know their health history, and what will we do with them while we're at the lake?" Then came the famous last words: "When the time is right, I promise we'll get some kittens."

The kid trying to find a home for his copycats swiveled his eyes up from the now empty box to Teresa and Mikkel and said, "If I don't find these kittens a home today, my dad says he's going to put them to sleep." I knew it was over. "Scoot over, Scooter," I said as we left with two new Beckers: Turbo and Tango.

My impulse adoption story has a good ending. For years, Turbo and Tango have happily served with distinction on rat patrol in our barn. But for many people, giving into the impulse to bring home a cute little kitten or puppy brings on disaster. Nature intended for the young in any species to be irresistible as a form of protection. One look at a puppy or kitten, and we can fall right into nature's trap with our hearts in overdrive and our heads in emergency brake mode. Our emotions say yes, and our brains don't consider the full impact of a fifteen-year or so commitment of daily responsibilities and annual expenses. Typically, we fall into love and take home that unexpected puppy or kitten with no advance planning or preparation for life with the adult pet. So when the relationship begins to go downhill due to house soiling, scratching, digging, excessive barking, not using the litter box, or rowdy behavior, we are inclined to respond impulsively once again, to rid ourselves of the unexpected headaches.

Six million unwanted companion animals are surrendered to shelters every year. We send our pets to death row for the crime of being unwanted or a nuisance. Unruly behaviors that contribute to these family breakups, in most cases, could have been easily prevented and with time—and the right kind of attention—corrected.

Purebred animals are not immune from this death sentence. My veterinary colleagues and I have battled the medical and personality problems of irresponsible breeding fueled by hit movies and television shows. Examples of these popular breeds are German shepherds (*Rin Tin Tin*), collies (*Lassie*), cocker spaniels (*Lady and the Tramp*), and more recently goldens (*Air Bud*), Dalmatians (*101*), and Jack Russell terriers (Eddie on *Frasier*). We cringe at the thought of the next pet fad, knowing that amateur breeding can release the recessive medical and behavioral problems of any breed.

As you can see, we need to do more than window-shopping in selecting a future long-term, four-legged companion. Just like dating, selecting a pet is about more than just good looks. We need to get past the physical attraction, analyze our compatibility, and be sure we are ready to make a commitment. Otherwise, we may fall into irreconcilable differences and the heartache of a family breakup. My hope is to show you how to make this decision wisely—with equal parts love and logic—so you can find a loving partner to share your life with no matter what your condition, illness, or need.

Are You Pet-Ready?

AS PSYCHOLOGISTS HAVE TOLD US for years, before we are ready to enter into a healthy, loving relationship, we must be comfortable with who we are and define what we want. To get a better handle on your critical pet relationship needs and desires, answer the following questions:

1. Do I have time for the daily feeding, loving, playing, training, and exercising of a pet?

2. Can I cover the cost of veterinary care, pet insurance, training, pet food, boarding, grooming, and pet supplies in my monthly budget?

3. Am I strong enough to properly train and manage a large, active adult dog? Do I have any physical or housing limitations that may make it difficult, if not impossible, to walk a dog regularly?

4. Am I restricted by my living situation on the size or type of pet?

5. Does anyone in my family show signs of allergies to fur or pet dander?

6. If I am planning to add a cat to one or more at home, do I have enough space for each cat to prevent territorial fighting?

7. When I go on vacation, what will I do with my pet?

8. If I need to work long hours or be away from home for extended periods of time, how will I properly care for my pet?

If you are considering a pet other than a dog or cat, check out the free information available on alternative pets from the American Veterinary Medical Association. (Send a self-addressed, stamped envelope to The Veterinarian's Way of Selecting a Proper Pet, AVMA Literature Requests, 1931 N. Meacham Rd., Schaumburg, Illinois 60173–4360.)

Let's pull back the curtain a bit farther to help you imagine a pet in your world. For example, if you're a single person living in an apartment and working fourteen hours a day, you may want a dog that doesn't nuisance-bark during the day, but who will still bark appropriately if something goes bump in the night. Or if companionship rather than protection is your motivation, with that many hours out of the house, a cat might be a better choice.

Do you want a big, lumbering, goofy kind of dog, or a small, meteoric, smart one? Do you want a dog with a huggable coat, or one with a short, bristly coat that doesn't leave your clothes looking like you wear your pet to work? Should your cat be a rough-and-tumble kind of cat that can chase a length of silly string with the kids, or a bookshelf kind of cat that's the epitome of "eye candy"?

To develop pet-people matchmaking exercises, I asked for help from Dr. Rolan Tripp, a veterinary behavior consultant and an affiliate professor of animal behavior at Colorado State University College of Veterinary Medicine. He has developed what we call the Tripp Tests for Selecting a New Pet. Honest answers can help you narrow the field of possible pets. Of course it's not all just cold, hard logic. Picking out the right pet, just like picking out the right mate, is also about finding the magic . . . chemistry.

If you are willing to adopt a stray from the local animal shelter, and I hope you are, heed Dr. Tripp's step-by-step shelter pet selection guide. These selection tools only skim the surface of Dr. Tripp's vast arena of applied knowledge of the interactive world of people and pets. For more detailed information, consider tapping into Dr. Tripp's website: www. AnimalBehavior.net.

Matchmaking Service

To find your best pet match, I recommend that you first review these fifteen vital questions, then take the Tripp Tests that follow. As a point of explanation, the key words or phrases in parentheses after the subject titles—example (See Size) below—are cued to specific questions in the Tripp "Pet Selection" Tests. For example, if you take the Tripp Test to select the IdealDog™, and size is of a high priority, you can instantly refer back to number 1, "Size Matters," for more information.

1. SIZE MATTERS! *(See Size)*

When selecting a dog based on size, the first consideration is simple bulk. Remember: the bigger the dog, the bigger the cleanup! Another consideration in selecting size is life span. Larger dogs tend to mature more rapidly, but have shorter life spans than smaller breeds. Smaller dogs may save you dollars on the pet food bill, but can make up for it by needing more frequent professional dental care.

Be sure you picture that cute little puppy in his full adult size and personality. Know that the five-pound, smaller-than-a-breadbox rottweiler puppy that you can easily sling under your arm like a baby now will, in six months, be strong-arming you for attention with eighty-plus pounds of influence.

If one of your goals in getting a dog is physical protection, consider a large, dark-colored dog like that "rottie" for visual intimidation, but with a big dog, be prepared for a rigorous schedule of puppy and adult obedience training to prevent unruly and unwanted behaviors. If you prefer a smaller dog, a determined terrier type will sound the alarm with conviction. Terriers, like rottweilers, have strong wills, so both require early and ongoing training. If you don't teach terriers and other active, intelligent breeds what you want them to do, they tend to create their own job descriptions. For example, rat terriers and beagles will burrow, basset hounds will bellow, border collies will round up their toys, and Labs will swim laps in the pool.

If a lap lounger and cuddle bug is more your style, consider a smaller, calmer, fluffier breed such as a papillon or Maltese. Pugs are a small breed that can be easily trained, are good with children, and more about fun and games. Havanese, Maltese, Lhasa apsos, shih tzus, and poodles are more laid back than the terriers and do not shed, but they do require regular grooming.

Do long legs, bedroom eyes, or luscious lips turn you on? Just remember that the longer the legs on the dog you select, the longer the walk or run you need to provide daily. Those bedroom eyes may melt your heart, but bloodhound eyes also catch more dust, debris, and infections, so grab your pocketbooks. Be prepared for those large, luscious lips—of Newfoundlands and St. Bernards—to give you extra slurpy kisses and to slime your environment. It's a Kodak moment when those long, droopy basset hound or Old English sheepdog ears fall into the food or water bowl. But floppy-eared dogs are generally more prone to ear infections than those with erect ears. Dogs with erect ears tend to look more intimidating than their floppy-eared counterparts. Erect ears, like tails, can twitch with interest and wiggle in delight. As for the tail, a long, wagging beauty may be your cup of tea, but don't put that cup on the coffee table if you want it to be safe from a long tail's path of destruction.

2. SOME LIKE IT HOT! *(See Coat and Grooming)*

Some like it hot, but not your long- or double-coated pet friend that was intended to pull a sled in snow country! Will your pet live inside or outside most of the time? What are the extreme temperatures in your local climate? Will you be able to keep a short-coated pet warm or a thick-coated pet cool?

I was recently disheartened to see a longhaired, double-coated Samoyed panting and trying to keep cool in a steamy Miami locale. At the other extreme, at a mountain cabin I saw a Rodeo Drive high-fashion sweater on a Chihuahua that was still shivering and uncomfortable. Longer coats require more combing, brushing, and grooming expenses. Is your pocketbook prepared to take your poodle to the groomer every four to six weeks? I see exacting clients taking their house dogs to professionals for weekly baths, extended brush-outs, and toenail filings. This costs a pretty penny, but produces a beautiful look.

Don't be fooled into thinking that short-coated pets shed less than their long-coated counterparts. In general, the shorter the coat, the greater the shedding, because the hairs spend more time replacing themselves instead of growing longer. Any pet hair can trigger an allergic response. Cats like the Persian and dogs like the Samoyed have double coats with a top layer of hair that sheds continuously, as well as a fine undercoat. Some say double-coated breeds are more likely to cause allergic reactions, as they release more dander with the shedding. With regard to the color of the coat, consider matching the pet's color to the color of flooring in your home to help camouflage shedding.

3. AGES AND STAGES *(See Age)*

Adopting a puppy is like starting out with a blob of soft, wet clay. It will be easier for you to mold the personality and habits during the critical learning period between two and four months old when your puppy's brain is like a sponge. If you enroll your three-month-old pup into an off-leash, puppy socialization and training class, you can significantly reduce aggression, increase playfulness, and enhance Bonding to your family and other pets.

With that said, there are advantages to maturity. Adopting an adult dog offers worthy pluses. What you see is what you get! His personality is already established, and can be temperament tested more reliably than a young puppy. Just like an economy car, young adult dogs can be less expensive and get good mileage. The cost of puppy vaccines and altering is typically behind you. If they were indoor dogs, you won't need to invest as much time in house-training them. A young adult dog may have many good years ahead, but beware of unwanted "baggage"—existing behavioral or medical problems—that may have led to their being available for adoption. Like reaching for the ripest fruit higher up in the tree, you take some risk!

Don't rule out adopting a senior pet. Both cats and dogs in their golden years tend to be more easily contented and calm—the perfect companion for a kicked-back kind of dude or a lady who likes her leisure time to be low-key. Just be sure you put enough money in the piggy bank. Like cars with lots of miles, pets in their geriatric years may require unexpected and more costly maintenance in the form of teeth cleaning, ear, eye, and skin care, and thorough annual exams that include blood work, radiographs, and lifetime medications.

4. SEX MATTERS (See Gender)

In general, fighting, roaming, and urine marking are more common with intact male (unsterilized) dogs or cats. Intact female dogs and cats can develop medical problems and cancers related to their reproductive systems. An intact female cat may drive you crazy with the look of love in an unseemly nonstop heat cycle of vocalization, rubbing, and rolling. Intact dogs may spot blood on your favorite white rug during the few days twice yearly when they undergo a heat cycle. Unless you sport a passion for breeding to protect the integrity of the breed in best of looks, health, and behavior, I *strongly* urge you to spay or neuter your pet. This is important not just to reduce the risk of medical and behavioral problems, but also to help reduce the overpopulation of homeless dogs and cats. Once the pet is neutered, the personality difference between male and female has been essentially "neutralized."

5. PEOPLE PLEASERS (See People Orientation)

Just like us, there are pets who simply love to party! Those same pets struggle with their alone time. Social butterfly dogs may chew, dig, bark, or whine to relieve their anxiety while waiting for their people-fix and the action to begin again. These dogs just long to be close to you!

If dogs or cats are not raised around children, they may not want to give kids the time of day, or worse, may become high-strung, snappy, or scratchy. Never leave a young child and an unfamiliar dog unattended. Make sure all contact between youngsters and pets is supervised to avoid pets being mistreated. Teach children to be kind and gentle with pets. Show a small child how to ask a dog to sit and then give it a dog cookie. Bribery will get you everywhere!

Which dogs make good gym junkies? If you spend your leisure time with sneakers on and your idea of fun is a good run, consider the sporting (retrievers, setters, pointers, spaniels, or perhaps a vizsla or weimaraner) or working breeds (akita, malamute, boxer, shepherd, Doberman, Great Dane, rottweiler, or Great Pyrenees). They tend to be high-energy dogs, and can keep up with you on a bike ride or jog. Make sure you work them up to it gradually—condition them—if you are seeking mini-marathon status.

Although work- and sport-oriented, these breeds have the brains and aptitude for learning that can make training sessions more fun for both of you. If you are successful in gaining a leadership ranking in their eyes, they will live to please you.

If you are looking for a Velcro pet, one that prefers sticking close to you more than playing with his toys or pet brothers and sisters, consider this personality test prior to adoption. In a neutral, enclosed environment, after holding or playing with the pet, simply put it down and move away. If the pet follows you, consider that a good sign of social interest. If the pet ignores you or moves away from you, you may be in the company of a future shrinking violet or dog that doesn't agree that no man is an island. If the pet play-attacks your leg, nips at your heels, or grabs your pant leg, you may be witnessing the first signs of a future prizefighter. Be forewarned!

---

6. ROOMMATES *(See Pet Orientation)*

Does your current pet really want or need a four-legged pal? Could you be accused of taking your pet's feelings for granted? The truth of the matter is that not all cats or dogs want to share their homes with a stranger, and will resist dividing up the home turf, toys, and affection. When your cat rubs her face on the couch or corner of the door, she is planting the equivalent of a stake, claiming her territory.

Cats are not instinctively pack animals because they don't hunt in groups. Just because your cat is lonely for you during the day, that doesn't mean she wants competition for your attention when you are home. Cats that don't want to share their abode may start spraying smelly urine warning signs around the house to make it perfectly clear to the intruder who was there first. Dogs don't do well when they are treated as equals. We need to learn and respect their pecking orders. It is also much harder for us to train two dogs, walk two dogs, or sometimes even feed two dogs at once.

With that said, if you do proceed to add a new pet to your household, here are a few tips on how to create a successful first encounter. As they say, "You only have one shot at making a good first impression!" First, if possible, bring the dogs to meet in a neutral setting such as a dog park, beach, or kennel. This diffuses that argument of "whose house is it anyway?" Just like people, some dogs hit it off right away; others just don't seem to have good chemistry.

When introducing a new cat to the family, begin temporarily with the newcomer in a separate room, like a bathroom, for several days to allow for a gradual introduction. Feed the cats on either side of a closed door so they can associate a positive experience with the whiff of each other blended in. Consider rubbing the same towel over each hair coat so that their scents intermingle as a strategy to reduce hissing hostilities.

In both cases, whether introducing a new dog or cat, give the resident pets the privileges of rank. Greet the senior pet first, feed him first, allow him in the most rooms or places in the house (ranging from your lap to your bed), and give him the most attention. That pet has earned it.

7. GETTING TO KNOW YOU *(See Vocal/Territorial Traits)*

Some pets simply have more to say than others. Vocalization can result from design or from environmental cues. Hunting breeds bay or howl to alert hunters to their location. Breed specifics are why beagles bugle and shelties shout! Dogs such as shelties, miniature schnauzers, and German shepherds are bred to sound the bark alarm against intruders. Sometimes these dogs just like to hear the sound of their own voices. Sound like anybody you know?

If you have neighbors within earshot, an excessive yapper may jeopardize good neighbor relations. Just as there are people who talk on the phone to relieve stress, there are dogs who bark to relieve their stress from being home alone, bored, uncomfortably hot or cold, itchy, sore, untrained, underexercised, or stressed by children who tease, possums that walk the fence, or cats that dare to invade their backyards. If you are the kind of person who wants your pet to be a good listener while you do all the talking, you might try this test before selecting a dog. Bounce a ball, squeak a toy, hold up an irresistible treat, jump up and down, and see how excited and how easy it is to get the dog to bark and how long it lasts.

On the other hand, if you prefer two-way conversations, you can develop your pet's vocal talents by answering their cries and responding to them with food, petting, or undivided attention. What gets rewarded gets repeated! If you enjoy conversing with your feline friend, consider selecting a breed that is genetically wired to be a big talker, such as the Siamese, Balinese, and Tonkinese cats. The quieter breeds generally have heavier, hairier builds and include the Persian and Maine coon.

---

8. ESPRESSO ANYONE? *(See Activity Level)*

How can one resist the pet in the litter that is the most animated and eager for your attention? If you are highly active, then this selection may be right for you. However, if activity at the end of a long day gets on your nerves and you prefer peace and quiet most of the time, then look for a match to your personality. The puppy that is slow to warm up and waits patiently for you to approach may be the low-key friend that will share a quiet evening of classical music and a good book in the garden with you. Remember hearing that a tired child is a well-behaved child? If you are unable to jog his heebie-jeebies (nervous energy) out, your dog may act like a Mexican jumping bean when you'd prefer a real live Beanie Baby lying on the beanbag chair with you. Keep your active dog busy or he may find work you didn't know you needed done, like recycling your backyard soil or turning that table leg into sawdust. Active pets are more likely to create their own activity, such as chewing on our shoes, if we do not provide enough mental or physical stimulation. When an active dog starts digging holes to find China, they aren't trying to spite us: They are simply attempting to pass the time or burn off nervous energy like we do when we chew our fingernails, pace, or pop our knuckles. Sadly, many people aren't very patient and usually consider these to be unwanted behavior problems that are difficult to control, and that may warrant removing the dog from the home.

Unless you are an athlete looking for an *Air Bud*, a cowboy looking for a dog to run your herd, or a dog trainer heading for obedience trials, think twice before selecting a dog from the hunting and sporting breeds. Rather, consider a calmer dog with a low-to-moderate activity. Great Danes and greyhounds are two of the calmer large breed dogs. Greyhound rescue groups visit pet stores nationwide. Do not choose a greyhound if you have any thoughts of spending time with an off-leash dog. Many greyhounds don't look back when they take off after that squirrel or cat.

9. NERVOUS NELLIES *(See Excitability)*

Excitability is slightly different from activity level. An excitable pet may be calm as long as you don't hit the trigger. If something strange, new, or fun pops into sight, look out! These dogs may launch into animated displays of barking, jumping, spinning, and running that make it difficult to find their off switch. An easily excitable pet may become distracted during training. Pets with calm personalities generally demonstrate longer attention spans, which makes them easier to train.

10. GIRLS JUST WANT TO HAVE FUN *(See Playfulness)*

To rank a pet on the Play-O-Meter, bring along toys to use in making your selection. Cats get Play-O-Meter points by chasing a toy, pouncing on it, or batting it with their paws. When meeting your potential kitty, wiggle or drag a string in front of her or toss a mouse-size object into the kennel and watch what she does. Dogs get points for chasing or picking up a toy in their mouths, play bows, perky ears, and wagging tails. Bounce a ball or squeak a toy in front of the puppy and see how he responds. Speak to him in an upbeat, jolly tone; clap your hands; crouch down and pat the floor and see if the pooch pounces back in a playful fashion.

Cats or dogs in unfamiliar surroundings may be too stressed to give you a good indication of their play aptitudes. Be patient. This pet may be wonderful, but just not exert himself on a first date. If possible, spend extended periods of time with the pet in a calm environment until he relaxes enough to let you see him for who is really is and what makes him tick. If the pet insists on being a party pooper and playfulness is important to you, move on.

11. STAR PUPILS *(See Training)*

Dogs thrive on routine and consistent house rules. If you are looking for an Einstein elkhound or a professor poodle that can master advanced types of commands, you'll need a dog that scores high in attention span, desire to please, and intelligence.

Smart dogs can become know-it-alls. Certainly, brains make training sessions more successful. Intelligence without proper training can drive a dog to take over a household. A dog with natural leadership tendencies may watch us serve him food, clean up his toilet area, pet or groom him like a subordinate might in the wild, and then assume he wears the pants in the family. Talk about ego!

To keep a dog securely in his place as a subordinate in the family, we need to show him consistently that we are in charge. A dog will follow our lead if he believes we are reliable, benevolent leaders and that he can trust us to provide for him if he simply follows our rules. Instead of freely putting down the food bowl, we must first ask the dog to sit or perform any other command as a reminder that nothing in life is free. If the dog pleases us by doing what we ask, then we reward the dog's obedience by feeding him. Before the dog gains any privilege such as going inside or outside, being stroked or given toys or playtime, we must first demonstrate our leadership in the household by asking the dog to do something to show loyalty and willingness to follow the leader. Before a dog will learn from us, he must be motivated by our status in relationship to his survival. Dogs naturally worship their leaders.

The dog must clearly know what it is we are asking him to do. We may be unaware of how confusing our signals are to our dogs. We may blame them for disobedience when in reality they are confused by our training methods. Attending a reputable obedience class can help us successfully communicate with our dogs and build the leadership relationship and structure our dogs need.

The length of a dog's attention span is one factor in his aptitude for learning that impacts successful training. To test this aptitude, first try to get his attention by taking a treat from in front of his nose up to your eyes and saying, "Watch me," in a high, animated voice. Use exaggerated facial gestures, mouth sounds, and eye movements to focus the dog on your face. Once the dog looks in your eyes, animate them even more, saying, "Good dog" in baby-talk tones. Observe how long the dog stays focused on you. If possible, give the dog the treat while he is still looking up at you, and repeat the sequence with a new treat. Be sure to compare several dogs in your matchmaking selection process.

---

12. MACHO, MACHO DOG! *(See Doggedness)*

Macho, macho dog; I wanna have a macho dog! Doesn't it seem likely that we would want a dog that is bold, strong, and "dogged"? We may feel more protection from a macho dog when, in fact, we may be more at risk. Overly confident, dominant personality dogs end up biting their owners more often than protecting them. If you have a strong nature, a desire to work daily with your dog on commands, and an ability to stay consistent with your house rules, then you may be able to manage a strong-willed, powerful dog. However, if you prefer to spoil your pets and are more of a spontaneous personality, then I recommend you select a more passive dog that is more naturally eager to please and accept commands and training without challenging you for leadership.

14. ONLY HER HAIRDRESSER KNOWS FOR SURE
(See Markings)

Do blondes have more fun? There are breeders, behaviorists, and veterinarians who suggest that the color of a cat's coat indicates certain personality traits.

For example, generally speaking, tabby cats are known to be highly social, affectionate, and able hunters. Solid black cats are considered even-tempered, intelligent, and friendly. On the other hand, you might be advised not to introduce a new kitten to your calico or tortoise shell cat, as she doesn't take kindly to having her routines changed or sharing her queen status and kingdom with others. Just ask your veterinarian if they prefer to examine a calico or a tabby. There are veterinarians who view tricolored cats as temperamental and aggressive. This does not even scratch the surface, as there are many registered cat breeds with specific coat colors and pattern variations. For example, is a Somali easier-going than an Abyssinian? Does a Siamese talk more than a Burmese? Let's not get started. These are fighting words among those who genuinely care about the unique qualities of specific breeds of cats. A discussion on this topic by serious breeders could dwarf most political debates in comparison!

There are lies, damn lies, and statistics. Let's look at statistics. White cats and dogs, especially those with blue eyes, are likely to lose their hearing over time. A recent report given at the annual conference of the American Academy of Allergy, Asthma, and Immunology showed that dark-hued kitties were two to four times more likely to trigger moderate or severe sneezing and wheezing with patients than fair-haired felines.

15. KEEP THAT MOTOR RUNNING! *(See Vocal/Purrs)*

I don't think there's such a thing as too much purring. The more your cat purrs like a Mack truck on the open highway the better, since the sound of a cat purring warms our hearts and makes us smile. Putting your ear on the chest of a purring cat feels as basic as a baby listening to her mother's heartbeat. How can you test a cat for her tendency to purr easily and often? When you pick the kitty up, does she rev up her engine and keep it humming while she is being held and loved? Can you hear her purr from across the room? Can you feel her motor running when you put your hand on her chest? As a rule of thumb, the more easily a cat purrs, the more she will seek your attention, follow you around, and set up housekeeping in your lap. If you want to pass time with your kitty, select a purr machine. I feel a siesta coming on!

Looking for Love in All the Right Places

NOW IT'S TIME TO GET down to the nitty-gritty to help you select and fine-tune the type of dog or cat that will best suit you. We'll use the Tripp Tests for Selecting a New Pet to reveal your every whim and desire. If you share your household with others, hand out copies of these tests and compare results. Rank the following traits as low, medium, or of high priority. Ready? Let's begin!

Tripp Test for Selecting a New Dog

BODY PRIORITY

(In each category, mark L, low priority; M, medium importance; or H, closest to my IdealDog ™)

SIZE:

__teeny-weeny   __pint-size   __knee-high   __waist-high
__the bigger the better

COAT:

___short and smooth   ___soft and fluffy   ___long with feathers   ___wiry   ___curly
___double-coated

MARKINGS:

___one solid color   ___patterned/brindled   ___multicolored

GROOMING:

shedding: ___none   ___moderate   ___heavy   ___needs regular brushing
___needs regular haircuts

AGE:

___pup less than six months old   ___pup six months to one year old
___adult two to six years old   ___senior more than six years old

GENDER:

___intact male   ___neutered male   ___intact female   ___spayed female

MIND PRIORITY
(In each category, mark L, low priority; M, medium importance; or H, closest to my IdealDog ™)

PEOPLE ORIENTATION:

___independent   ___people-pleaser   ___social butterfly   ___Velcro buddy

PET ORIENTATION
(toward other house pets):

___lover   ___good friends   ___antisocial   ___hostile

VOCAL/TERRITORIAL TRAITS:

___barks rarely   ___barks, stops quickly   ___barks moderately   ___very vocal

ACTIVITY LEVEL:

___super athlete   ___weekend warrior   ___strolls in the park   ___laps around yard
___couch potato

EXCITABILITY:

___jumping bean   ___hot potato   ___short fuse   ___slow burn   ___no pulse

PLAYFULNESS:

___Toys R Us   ___only on weekends   ___work before pleasure   ___party pooper

TRAINING:

___show dog   ___working dog   ___house dog   ___problem-free dog   ___wild dog

DOGGEDNESS:

___strong-willed   ___independent   ___team player   ___passive

Tripp Test for Selecting a New Cat

Here's a creative assessment test devised by Dr. Tripp to help you find a fine feline friend.

BODY PRIORITY
(In each category, mark L, low priority; M, medium importance; or H, closest to my IdealCat ™)

S I Z E :

___petite   ___average   ___big and tall

C O A T :

___short   ___fluffy ___long

M A R K I N G S :

___one solid color   ___patterned   ___two color ___tricolored

G R O O M I N G :

___self-grooming   ___moderate brushing   ___requires professional routine

A G E :

___kitten   ___adult   ___senior

G E N D E R :

___intact male   ___neutered male   ___intact female   ___spayed female

MIND PRIORITY
(In each category, mark L, low priority; M, medium importance; or H, closest to my IdealCat ™)

P E O P L E   O R I E N T A T I O N :

___hide 'n' seek   ___independent   ___a greeter   ___lap addict

P E T   O R I E N T A T I O N :

___aloof   ___hostile   ___buddies

V O C A L S / M E O W S :

___mute   ___greeter   ___never ending story

V O C A L S / P U R R S :

___minor key   ___major symphony   ___silence is golden

P L A Y F U L N E S S

___ring around the rosy   ___catch as cat can   ___snooze alarm

R E A C T I V I T Y :

___invisible cat   ___slightly curious   ___wait for me!

I Pick the Perfect Pet for Lilly

Early in my veterinary career, I met Lilly. She became a favorite client of mine. After the loss of her beloved pet, it took many years before she could think about adopting another one. In sizing up Lilly's indomitable spirit, I wholeheartedly recommended that she select a black Labrador retriever just like Luke, the dog I had as a boy.

Unfortunately, I made this recommendation solely on my Lab loyalty, not on my knowledge of how Lilly's needs, abilities, and lifestyle matched the breed characteristics of a Labrador.

If I'd taken the time to ask questions, I might have learned that Lilly was battling severe arthritis and found simple movements, such as hair brushing, difficult. I might have also discovered that Lilly was prone to falls due to vertigo, that she was allergic to pet dander, and that her immaculate home was full of antique furniture.

You can imagine my pride upon learning that Lilly had adopted a black Lab puppy and named him Cole (as in a black piece of coal). Veterinarians only partly jest when they say that Labradors "chew, 'til they're two and shed, 'til they're dead." True to form, Cole viewed Lilly's priceless furniture legs as convenient chew sticks. His fur flew during his fun romps in the house, causing Lilly to sneeze and wheeze through dozens of allergy inhalers. By age six months, Cole was forty pounds of wiggling muscle. He yanked on the leash like it was taffy as Lilly maneuvered her hurting hips through her antiques on the way to Cole's nightly walk. And instead of a fierce protector, Cole happily welcomed every doorbell-ringing stranger with an instant wagging tail.

Faced with difficult problems that were beyond her control, Lilly was forced to find Cole a more suitable home in the country. I learned a powerful lesson at the expense of this fine lady. After taking a careful profile of Lilly's wants, needs, and lifestyle, I made a second—and this time—lifelong match. Lilly traded in the heartache with Cole for a love affair with Miss Clairol, a homeless Devon Rex cat we had at the veterinary hospital. Miss Clairol (named because of the cat's characteristic kinky hair that sheds very little) loved curling up beside Lilly on the couch, watching sitcoms or reading late into the night. As it turned out, Lilly didn't need a guard dog to protect her from strangers. She needed a calm, caring cat to protect her against a far greater threat: loneliness.

If I had been able to give Lilly the Tripp Test, she would have been protected from my partisanship. You've heard love is blind. That's true for our pets and us. It is understandable that we develop a loyalty to a breed based on memories of a favorite pet. Passionate, responsible breeders who are dedicated to furthering the best qualities in their breed are known for giving objective information about the breed they promote. Their advice regarding selection of that breed will include the joys and the challenges you can expect. However, for mainstream America, we see our favorite breeds through rose-colored glasses. When it comes to discussing the best breeds of dogs, people have strong opinions based on their personal experiences. When looking for a good breed match for your life, don't confuse your neighbors' or family members' opinions with facts. Go to a reliable source. Check the Internet for information by AKC breed clubs or ask your veterinarian about the size, required care, and personality traits of different dogs. If you want the statistics about which dog breeds are most likely to raise your insurance rates because of their history of costly dog bite claims, call your home insurance agent.

In addition to the reference section provided in the back of this book, I highly recommend that you sort your way through your Tripp Test results with your trusted local veterinarian.

Many people think a modern veterinary hospital only offers medical and surgical services. When I graduated from veterinary school in 1980, pet selection, socialization, and behavioral training were not even a small blip on the veterinary practice Richter scale. We thought these issues distracted us from our focus on surgery and medicine. House soiling and other destructive behaviors were for dog trainers, not doctors, to solve. Not any more.

Today, an animal behavior class at a veterinary school or conference is often standing room only, and many veterinary hospitals have shelves brimming with behavior reference and resource materials. In addition to breed advice, the veterinarian can connect you to reputable breeders, shelters, and trainers.

Your veterinarian may give you a referral to a veterinary behaviorist. This relatively new profession offers the advanced training and network to help you select the best pet up front or to help you navigate through any incompatibilities you are experiencing with your pet. Veterinary behaviorists are qualified to assist you in redirecting any bad habits your pet has developed that might otherwise jeopardize your relationship and diminish the Bond you share.

When you have narrowed your choice to a particular breed, visiting some of the websites at the back of the book can help you determine the costs over a life span. These websites also highlight some of the medical and behavioral problems that are typical of different breeds, so that you go into this long-term commitment with your eyes fully opened.

SELECTING AN ADULT DOG AT A SHELTER

Dogs with great personalities and potential can be found at your local shelter. Dr. Tripp shares his strategy to help you scan the "heart-tugging" landscape of shelter cages for a dog that will complement your lifestyle. The common denominators found in good dogs include a calm instead of hyperactive nature, a friendly attitude toward people and pets, and a basic intelligence grounded in a stable attention span. Here is how to recognize these redeeming qualities.

1. Walk down each row of available kennels. Observe your first impressions to see if you have an immediate "connection" with any particular pet. Watch what the dogs do as you walk past the kennels. Look for dogs that want to come closer and take a good look at you with friendly body postures and eyeballs. Rule out dogs that are frantically jumping around in their kennels or show signs of aggression.

2. Approach the kennel with a potential candidate and act as calmly as possible. Stand relaxed and shift your weight to one foot. Look in the direction of the dog, but avoid direct eye contact. Ideally, what you are looking for is a dog that approaches you, looks up with interest, then sits to show submission. A small amount of vocalization is acceptable, but not excess whining or barking. Look for a moderate amount of eye contact as a sign of intelligence and eagerness to please. Although perfectly good dogs may be eliminated by these observations, seeing these qualities gives you a good start on making the best selection possible.

3. Select dogs that are at a minimum of four months of age to reduce the risk of life-threatening illnesses that can spread through well-intentioned but overpopulated shelters.

4. If you have more than one good candidate, you may wish to test the dog's "reactivity." While still outside the kennel, suddenly raise your hands over your head, and slightly lunge forward toward the dog. If the dog reacts too aggressively back at you, he may not have an easygoing, stable disposition and may become a handful. If he moves away in slight fear, immediately drop the act and go to the next test.

5. Now act as friendly as possible as if to say, "I was just kidding. I would really like to be friends." Crouch down, talk in a happy voice, slap the ground or your leg, and encourage the dog to come to you. If the dog will not forgive the reactivity test, it is possibly too fearful to make a good pet. If he forgives you and willingly approaches you, he remains a candidate.

6. Ask the shelter staff if you can take out a few candidates, one dog at a time. Once the dog is out of its kennel and settles down, you are ready to see if the dog shows interest in you or ignores you to investigate his surroundings.

7. Evaluate the dog's activity level when he is out of the kennel compared to how he acted inside the kennel. It is normal to pull on a leash and jump excitedly when first let out of the kennel. However, if he continues unabated, this dog may be more work than you want or can handle. Look for a dog that is calm most of the time but becomes excited when appropriate.

8. Spend at least two minutes with each candidate to get a glimpse of his personality as he calms down. Look for an overall gentle, people-pleasing personality. Avoid dogs that demonstrate fearful or dominant personalities.

9. Pet the dog over his head and down his back. Determine if the dog likes to be touched and solicits more, or if he ignores your touch and tries to pull away. For the dogs craving your touch, pet his coat against the grain to see if he becomes upset or readily accepts it.

10. Walk the dog on a leash past the kennels of other dogs. Watch to see if the response to other dogs is aggressive, overly fearful, playful, or indifferent. In general, it is best to choose a "dog-friendly" dog, since one of any dog's greatest joys is hanging with and playing with other dogs during their life with you.

SELECTING AN ADULT CAT AT A SHELTER

If you're looking for a cat chum, Dr. Tripp shares his seven-step feline selection guide:

1. Walk through and simply look at every cat that is available for adoption. Observe your first impression to see if you have an immediate "love at first sight" experience. Based on this first pass, determine which cats you wish to test.

2. Pay particular attention to the coat length, pattern, and condition. The longer the coat, the more grooming is needed. Many veterinarians feel that tabby cats (any color) tend to be more loving and better hunters, therefore more playful, while calico cats are less flexible. In general, the attraction to a particular color or pattern is personal preference.

3. Stand outside of each cage housing a potential cat candidate. See if the cat recognizes and acknowledges your presence. Avoid fearful cats. At first, many cats will hiss but settle down after several seconds when they realize you pose no threat. Look for a cat that approaches the front of the kennel and seeks your attention and affection.

4. Try the "lovey eyes" test to see if a cat responds. Stand outside the kennel, relax your body, and half close your eyes the way cats do when they are very relaxed. Talk to the pet in gentle murmuring, like a gentle purring "kitty, kitty, kitty" and avoid any *S* sounds since hissing is a threat. If the cat responds by rubbing up against the cage or putting a paw through to make contact, consider her a candidate.

5. Bring a cat toy like a string or something that might elicit play. A playful cat is entertaining, and easier to exercise indoors with toys. Be aware that active young cats may also be more likely to climb curtains, shred furniture, and climb bookshelves, knocking over expensive household items.

6. Seek permission from the shelter staff to take the finalists out of their cages one at a time in a safe, enclosed area. Attempt to hold the cat, and observe if the cat accepts human companionship, or simply tries to get away.

7. If the cat can be held easily, observe for purring. How quickly does the cat purr? How loud? How long? Does the cat seem to be grateful for your attention and accept your handling? If so, you are holding a potential IdealCat™ buddy. In general, the more purring the better the personality.

CONCLUSION

Whew! As you can tell after going through these matchmaking tests, there is much more to picking a dog or a cat than first impressions, talking to a neighbor over the fence for his opinions, or gut instincts. These tests aren't designed to grade you, but rather work for you—and your future pet companion—so that your Bond can be beautifully strong and loving right from the start.

Filling the Perfect Pet Prescription

THE PERFECT PET PRESCRIPTION TO enhance your life and meet your unique needs is not easy. In fact, formulating it requires patience, homework, and teamwork. Armed with good information, you'll be more likely to achieve the perfect partnership, a fit where the needs of both pets and people are met. In this section, let me share with you the remarkable story of Darlene and Shadow; a perfect example of where a person's wants and needs were matched to the perfect pet by careful study and the help of professionals. And then let's take a look at some common medical conditions that present their own challenges and hear what leading medical experts have to say about the value of pets for the health and happiness of their patients.

Shadow: Darlene's Four-Legged Sentinel, Savior, and Soul Mate

Darlene Werremeyer divides her life into two phases: the pre-Shadow period and the life-with-Shadow period.

Darlene's health began deteriorating in 1991. Undiagnosed diabetes had narrowed her arteries, causing blockages to form. In 1997, she nearly died when an artery ruptured after a failed angioplasty procedure. In January 1998, she suffered a stroke that paralyzed her vocal cords and made speaking difficult. With her condition stabilized, Darlene joined her husband, Jon, at a family reunion in Yakima, Washington, where she met a miniature schnauzer named Maggie who belonged to Jon's grandmother. Darlene noticed that whenever Maggie was near, she felt calmer and talked more easily.

After returning from the reunion, Darlene told her neurologist, Dr. David Greeley, about the pet-induced tranquility she felt when near Maggie. Dr. Greeley told Darlene about studies he'd read about the role pets can play in reducing stress. Dr. Greeley wrote a prescription for her to get a dog.

After consulting with Dr. Greeley and upon doing extensive research at the library and online about temperament, cost of care, shedding, and trainability, they decided a miniature schnauzer would be just what the doctor ordered. On the recommendation of a veterinarian, they visited a reputable breeder, Judy Zimmerman, who helped Darlene pick out the perfect puppy, the runt of the litter, when he was only five days old. For weeks Judy accommodated Darlene visiting her little partner until the day of her birthday, when Jon took Darlene to pick up the now-weaned puppy she promptly named Shadow. This puppy quickly demonstrated his "dog smarts" by becoming house-trained in three days and mastering "sit," "stay," "shake hands," "roll over," "beg," and "bow" with relative ease.

But Shadow's true talents emerged when he was six months old. It was two days before Christmas and Darlene, feeling fatigued, decided to take a rest on the sofa. Shadow kept pawing at her arm, whining and staring at the blood monitor machine near the arm of the sofa. Finally, Darlene checked the machine and discovered that her blood sugar level was dangerously low.

This wasn't a one-time act. A month later, Shadow began to pester

Darlene, licking her in the face and not leaving her alone. After he gained her attention, he shifted his attention to the blood monitor machine. Darlene took another glucose test and confirmed that Shadow's strange insistence was no fluke. Shadow was alerting Darlene to plummeting blood sugar levels to prevent her from losing consciousness.

The Werremeyers worked with professional dog trainers to develop Shadow into an assistance dog who works as a "medic alert" service dog. Now when they go out, Shadow proudly wears his neon orange service dog vest, and Darlene carries a copy of Dr. Greeley's prescription for her.

Dr. Greeley, a lifetime dog lover, recognized that pairing Darlene with a dog could prove to be powerful medicine. "The fact that Darlene had a major stroke and hasn't had to visit my office in more than two years is strong validation that Shadow has worked wonders on her rehabilitation and her quality of life," says Dr. Greeley. A believer in the power of pets to heal, Dr. Greeley has prescribed dogs for people with epilepsy and depression, and advises patients with chronic or crippling pain to get a cat.

Before Shadow, diabetes sent Darlene to the emergency room three to four times a year in a crisis. Since Shadow, she's never had to be rushed to the hospital for low blood sugar. At first, Darlene's endocrinologist, Dr. Carol Wysham, was skeptical about the value of a dog for her condition, but she's come to appreciate what a positive effect Shadow's companionship has had on Darlene.

Although she still takes ten prescriptions a day, Darlene calls Shadow her "medical miracle" and a "blessing." "Shadow is the best medicine any doctor could prescribe," says Darlene. "If Shadow had been a pill that had produced this dramatic a difference in my life—physically, mentally, and socially—we would hail it as a miracle drug."

Pets and Their Vital Roles in Chronic Medical Conditions

Darlene is an example of someone who did everything right. She assessed her medical condition and her physical and economic limits. She worked with a veterinarian, her doctor, a breeder, and a trainer to choose a pet that blended perfectly into her life and met her needs. Shadow also added new dimensions of security and love to Darlene's life. Well-thought-out matches like this are happening every day. Here are just a few examples of pets that match up perfectly with a human medical condition.

ALLERGIES AND ASTHMA: AHHHHHH . . . . . . CHOOSE

Allergy to dogs or cats occurs in about 15 percent of the population. For people with asthma, nearly 30 percent are allergic to furry animals. But many allergy or asthma sufferers want or need pets. And contrary to many parents' instincts and doctors' beliefs, infants who grow up with cats or dogs may be less likely to suffer from allergies and asthma later in life, preliminary research suggests. "Traditionally, most people have thought that increased exposure to these allergens leads to more allergies," said Dr. Darryl Zeldin of the National Institute of Environmental Health Sciences. "But I think those conclusions are being reevaluated."

New evidence suggests that exposure to pets early in life might actually help the body build defenses against allergies and asthma, thereby protecting children from developing reactions, rather than triggering them.

"Kids exposed to animals seemed to be better off," said Christine C. Johnson, Ph.D., a senior research epidemiologist with the Henry Ford Health System in Detroit. Christine Johnson's study, which was presented at an American Thoracic Society Conference in 2001, tracked 833 children over seven years and found that exposure to two or more cats and dogs at one year of age made children less susceptible to other allergy-inducing substances by the time they turned seven, and that the exposure even improved some boys' lung functions.

Dr. Thomas Platts-Mills, an asthma and allergic disease specialist at the University of Virginia, runs a "cat" house there. His recent research published in *The Lancet* suggests that animals in the house (cats, in this case) can decrease the risk of asthma by causing humans to produce certain specialized helper cells that he says work as a form of tolerance. A team of Swedish researchers reached the same conclusion. But Platts-Mills cautions that cats aren't the only allergy triggers present. "We don't know if a cat's presence can decrease your risk for allergy to dust mites. A lot of children who are tolerant to cats are allergic to pollens." So the animal doesn't necessarily create a bulletproof shield against all things that trigger allergies and asthma.

Researchers say the new findings could be in line with what doctors call the "hygiene hypothesis." The theory holds that asthma and allergies have become increasingly common during the past three decades as family sizes have gotten smaller, standards of personal hygiene have risen, that a lack of environmental contaminants means that immune systems overreact when they encounter allergy- or asthma-producing substances. Other studies have shown that a rural lifestyle, residence on a farm or facility where animals are near the house, or the presence of dogs in the house protects against asthma. "We can't jump to conclusions," says Linda Ford, MD. "It might be too early to say this is protective."

For many allergy sufferers, dogs and cats are "just bearable" friends, whereas with asthma sufferers, these same pets can even be life-threatening.

Meet John. He's a lovely little pet. He likes to be held and stroked. Patients visiting Dr. Ford all know John. He lives in her office waiting room. John is a frog. He's not furry or feathery, because all of Dr. Ford's patients have allergies or asthma.

"We like to show patients alternatives," says Dr. Ford, former chairman of the American Lung Association. "Every pet doesn't have to be a dog or cat." In the "not feathery or furry" department, there are reptiles, such as iguanas, snakes, lizards, and salamanders and amphibians such as John the frog. Turtles, tropical fish, and hermit crabs can also make great pets for some kids and adults.

Keep in mind: "Cats seem to be more potent as far as triggering allergies and asthma than dogs," says Dr. Ford. And male cats shed more dander than female cats.

Cats with dark coats trigger two to four times more moderate or severe allergic responses in people than light-haired cats, according to researchers from Long Island College Hospital in Brooklyn, New York. They reported their study at the annual conference of the American Academy of Allergy, Asthma, and Immunology.

Contrary to popular belief, there is no such thing as a nonshedding, hypoallergenic pet. Every dog and cat creates dander, according to Dr. Ford, but you may react differently to different breeds. For her patients who insist on having a furry pet, Dr. Ford recommends a shorter-haired, smaller dog because there's "less dog" with less body surface and less hair to trap the dander. The smaller animal is easier to wash and groom—a practice she recommends be done every week.

AGING: WHEN YOUR MIND STARTS TO GO OR THE CLOCK STARTS TO SLOW

A hospital's long-term care unit adopted a large dog that, in turn, became quite attached to an aging gentleman with Alzheimer's disease. Because he was at a higher level of functioning, this resident was able to interact with the dog more than most. He would take the dog outside, play ball, and give him treats.

As the man's health declined and his mental abilities sunk deeper into the unknown world of Alzheimer's dementia, the man started to show agitation behaviors. One day, the man insistently began rattling the unit's locked door to the outside world. His frustration grew. The staff attempted to distract him. But the dog, in his own intuitive way, knew what to do. The dog quietly came up, grasped the man's shirt cuff in his mouth, and led the man gently back to his room.

Unlike some people, pets are unconditionally accepting of a person's limitations. "Dogs don't care what you look like or that you can't remember how to tie your shoes," says Kathy Richards, RN, Ph.D., a geriatrics researcher at the University of Arkansas for Medical Sciences. "Pets can provide that social contact that older people need."

Kathy Richards recalls a female Lab mix named Lady who lived in an Alzheimer's unit, a proven practice in the management of Alzheimer's patients that's becoming more accepted. Lady was the "live-in therapist" who enjoyed certain special occasions. The staff would periodically bring in a variety of petable pets, such as goats and lambs, even a full-grown sheep. This real-live petting zoo enlivened the hard-to-reach patients, some of whom could not communicate with words, but miraculously could interact socially with the animals.

Keep in mind: A compliant, friendly dog or cat (any breed, any size) can serve as another tool to help caregivers enhance quality of life. A puppy with sharp teeth is not the ideal pet for older people in this situation. Its teeth can easily tear an older person's naturally thinning skin. Watching goldfish provides a passive yet meaningful activity. Birds are also placed in nursing homes. Watching them fly around inside large cages, nesting, and feeding is far better than plopping people in front of televisions, says Kathy Richards.

ARTHRITIS: BIGGER IS NOT BETTER IF YOU HAVE ARTHRITIS

Arthritis comes in many forms. In fact, the Arthritis Foundation lists over one hundred different conditions under the umbrella of arthritis, from simple elbow pain or bursitis to severely disabling rheumatoid arthritis, osteoarthritis, fibromyalgia, and osteoporosis.

With arthritis, size *does* matter in selecting the right pet. Walking a big dog, for example, can be a pleasant exercise for someone with arthritis until the dog spots a squirrel and takes off with a shoulder and arm attached to the other end of the leash. Such stress can even trigger a flare-up of arthritis, according to Dr. Joel E. Rutstein, director of the Arthritis Diagnostic and Treatment Center in San Antonio.

Someone with frail bones because of osteoporosis must be vigilant about anything underfoot, including throw rugs or a cat. Dr. Rutstein suggests you weigh the companionship and psychological benefits against the hazards of falling over a pet and possible injury.

Keep in mind: A small dog. Dr. Rutstein's joy in life is his teacup Yorkie, Bebe—the perfect pet for someone with arthritis. She weighs in under the five-pound weight limit that Dr. Rutstein says someone with arthritis can comfortably lift.

Another benefit is exercise. Small pets, usually dogs, exert no force on sensitive shoulders, arms, and hands when walking on a leash. They won't be huffing and puffing you around the block. They like short walks, which are ideal for people with arthritis. Dr. Rutstein advocates that people with arthritis keep their hands limber by treating their pets to lots of petting.

"A dog or cat will usually allow you to rub their tummy all day long. You're thinking you're making the pet feel better, but in fact you are feeling better moving your hands. The fur and the feeling is very relaxing," says Dr. Rutstein, who considers this activity a form of self-hypnosis.

PET PROZAC: HEEL AND HEAL

Helen Curlee and Hillary, her Australian shepherd-husky mix, both have the painful form of degenerative arthritis known as osteoarthritis. At eighty pounds, too much for her stocky frame, Hillary needed to lose weight, according to her veterinarian, who recommended more and longer walks. And Helen also admitted she needed to shed some pounds. But exercise?

"Too boring," Helen said. "I've been overweight for a number of years, and have had arthritis since I was ten years old. I was not taking care of myself as my doctors had instructed me to do. I ate the wrong food, didn't exercise, and didn't lose the excess weight."

Helen didn't realize that the veterinarian was writing a pet prescription for her benefit, too. Helen and Hillary started walking twice daily around their Virginia apartment complex, which resulted in both of them shedding those unwanted pounds. Now birds of a feather, they both take the same arthritis medication and a low dose of daily aspirin.

"The thought that I was harming my dog made me look at myself and rethink my lifestyle," Helen says.

ADHD AND OTHER THINGS KIDS HAVE

Pets and kids—like bread and butter, they're a natural combination. That is, if the right pet is selected for the right child. No one wants to see an overly aggressive child trying to wrestle with a Chihuahua, or a black Lab knocking over a child with cerebral palsy. Children with emotional, behavioral, and health issues need careful consideration when selecting a compatible pet friend.

Big dog to the rescue: For hyperactive children, including those with attention deficit hyperactivity disorder (ADHD), there's merit in getting a dog—a big dog.

"Hyperactive kids are physical," says child psychologist Bunni Tobias, Ph.D., who has a private practice in southern California. "A big docile dog may be more tolerant to active play, especially when a little boy throws his body over the dog."

She encourages children to curl up with the big dog. Going tandem in this tactile setting soothes both the dog and the child. Just as when they were babies, children relax to heartbeats. The power of touch from hugging a gentle dog and feeling unconditional acceptance is a love that can mend a broken heart or quiet a troubled soul.

If you're thinking about giving your child a furry pet, however, Dr. Tobias advises parents to first rule out allergies, whose symptoms can look like hyperactivity behavior. Allergies cause kids to act out, be agitated, and have trouble paying attention—all signs of hyperactivity.

If a child has a history of harming pets, do not introduce a pet into the home (and certainly find a temporary home for the current family pet) until you have dealt with the reason the child is acting out. Get family counseling quickly. It's a mistake to subject a pet or a child to a potentially harmful relationship.

Lean on me . . . During a divorce or following a death, highly stressed children may act out and need someone to listen. Bunni Tobias suggests that a warm, furry friend can comfort children when the world is coming down around them. If children get overloaded easily and overreact by pushing, hitting, biting, and squeezing, they may not know their own strength and may hug with viselike grips. Obviously, she says a hamster, guinea pig, or bird would not live long around these children.

Children with mild neurological issues tend to overreact around animals. Dogs, for example, move rapidly and frighten them. When selecting a pet for these children, make your choice based on the animal's temperament, not his age. In this case, a feisty puppy may simply be too overwhelming. If selecting a pet from a shelter, Bunni Tobias recommends looking for a calm, controlled personality. Taking a dog trainer with you may be helpful in making the best choice.

Choose a cat as a perfect remedy for ill or weak children who may not have the energy to get down on the floor and play with a more active pet. A bedridden child or a child in a wheelchair may gain great joy from pulling a string for a kitten to chase. A well-chosen cat will curl up on a lap and lend a great deal of comfort to an isolated child. After all, it's a magical experience to be chosen by a cat! A child having difficulty sleeping may get a few extra winks soothed by the warm rhythms of a highly contented cat. Children with greater physical limitations might still be able to teach a bird to talk, or simply enjoy the enthusiasm of a bird responding to the attention they give it.

No matter which pet for which kind of child, Bunni Tobias suggests you help the relationship along by hiring a professional trainer. "Take the kid and the dog to a training class together," she says. "The child may be more motivated to learn from the trainer, even if the parents are giving him the same information."

CANCER: "WILL I OUTLIVE MY PET?"

Dr. Edward T. Creagan has treated more than fifty thousand patients for nearly thirty years at the Mayo Clinic, one of the country's premier medical centers. "There is no question that a pet adds a whole new dimension to the patient's remaining life," Dr. Creagan says. "Pets provide meaning and purpose to the lives of cancer patients during very stormy times. Optimists live longer than pessimists."

When your immune system is down due to cancer and chemotherapy treatment, you can stimulate natural cancer-killing cells if you are happy and at peace—two qualities pets bring to our lives. The clinical benefit of a furry friend at your bedside, as one part of a wide social support network, is a leap of faith. As Dr. Creagan says, "Anything is possible for those who believe."

Best pet: For an adult cancer patient undergoing rigorous treatment, a more sedate dog in his golden years is far more reasonable than a new Labrador puppy that is ready to chew through steel.

A high-strung small dog that demands nonstop attention may be as tiring to a cancer patient as a dog that requires a great deal of walking. Cancer patients need to take care of themselves first, and not have to worry about a pet that requires a rigorous exercise schedule. The ideal pet for a patient still gaining their strength back would be a low-maintenance pet, like a lap cat. Of course, there needs to be a plan for cat care while the owner is in the hospital for treatment or away all day for a chemo session.

DEPRESSION: MORE THAN PULLING A RABBIT OUT OF A HAT

He's a professional magician, but for pediatric psychologist Aubrey H. Fine, Ed.D., helping kids and adults with depression takes much more skill than pulling a rabbit out of a hat. Aubrey, however, does use a rabbit named Houdini in his practice, along with his three dogs, three cockatoos, lizards, a bearded dragon, and numerous fish.

The family pet can be part of a depressed person's support system, Aubrey explains. "The depressed person may be very alienated and alone, or may choose to be alone. An animal can get her out and involved."

Depression is one of the most common mental illnesses. Experts think actual clinical depression is caused by an imbalance in brain chemicals, notably serotonin. For vulnerable people, depression causes feelings of helplessness and hopelessness—much more than a simple case of the blues over a bad grade or a canceled date. Unfortunately, many people do not seek treatment. They may have been depressed for so long that they feel no hope or are too embarrassed to admit they may need mental health counseling.

Aubrey uses the Bond with animals to help his patients make remarkable recoveries. One young teenage girl was hospitalized for severe depression, he recalls, and was suicidal. The girl was keenly interested in animals, so Aubrey encouraged her to volunteer at a shelter. She did some dog walking, adopted kittens, and gradually recovered from her mental illness.

Especially in winter, when depression hits the hardest, a dog that needs to go outdoors can get someone with depression outside. And for people who would prefer indoor animals, a budgie or cockatiel can provide one-on-one indoor bonding.

DIABETES: LIFESAVING CANINE RESCUES MAKE SCENTS

Call it a sixth sense, but whatever you call it, the fact that a dog that can tell when your blood sugar is low is nothing short of incredible, and it is a possibly lifesaving miracle for someone with diabetes. For people with the more serious form of diabetes, called Type 1, low blood sugar (a condition called hypoglycemia) can be just a step away from passing out and possibly death.

As discussed earlier, possible clues to the dogs' perception may be that the owners sweat more during a low blood sugar episode or show muscle tremors. Perhaps the dogs respond to the owners' altered behavior patterns, common with low blood sugar.

HEART DISEASE: TRY THIS NATURAL BLOOD PRESSURE MEDICATION

The human heart is a sensitive barometer of our surroundings. And blood pressure is what James Lynch, Ph.D., Johns Hopkins professor and director of the Life Care Health Center in Baltimore, calls the "vascular seesaw of all human dialogue." He has observed that blood pressure rises when we speak to others, yet it falls when we relate to animals. Relating to our pet puts the body into the mode of hyperrelaxation—

creating "natural" blood pressure medication. His early research was among the first to document how petting lowers blood pressure.

While the pharmaceutical companies beat the drum for "quick fix" medicines for heart problems, James makes the case for pet therapy in classrooms. He wants to expose children to the contact, companionship, and communication among creatures in the living world. Heart disease starts when we are young. Imagine the power of early intervention into our children's health through the healing power of pets.

In one of his studies, Dr. Lynch found that when children were reading a book, their blood pressures went down when a pet was in the room. Just in the room. The children didn't even necessarily have to be relating to the animal for researchers to see the blood pressure–lowering effect of its presence.

Keep in mind: While scientific studies have repeatedly demonstrated you stand a much better chance of surviving one year after a heart attack if you own a pet, the best pet for a cardiac patient is a dog. Dogs demand regular, moderate exercise, something that is vital to a healthy heart. Both dogs and cats offer the wonderful benefit of aiding in stress reduction, but the best overall cardiac rehabilitation tool is a dog.

LIKE HEART ATTACKS, PETS CAN PREVENT A BRAIN ATTACK

"Medicine tends to focus on the high-tech, dramatic elements to treat stroke, such as major surgery and medicines," said Dr. David Wiebers, professor of neurology and chair of the Department of Cerebrovascular Diseases at the Mayo Clinic Stroke Center. "That's all well and good, but the impact of less dramatic, lifestyle-oriented prevention, including the role of animals, has been underemphasized."

Strokes are the third leading cause of death in America, and the leading cause of disability. If you suffer a stroke, fast action in getting to a hospital, and ideally to a stroke trauma team, may improve your outcome. Certain clot-busting drugs, if given within precious hours for clot-type strokes, can be truly life saving. But the best lifesaving outcomes of all are preventative measures, and pets play a role in reducing a major stroke risk factor: stress. The effects of stress can show up as high blood pressure, among other biological signs.

The impact of animals, for example, as low-tech prevention, "will be a lot greater on society than any of the high-tech interventions we've developed," Dr. Wiebers says, adding he believes that the right pet-and-person relationship can help prevent a stroke. "Research has shown that interacting with a companion animal can lower blood pressure and heart rate and reduce anxiety. It can also improve mood," observes Dr. Wiebers, author of *Stroke-Free for Life: The Complete Guide to Stroke Prevention and Treatment.*

Keep in mind: According to Dr. Wiebers, someone with severe limitations would benefit more from a passive, low-maintenance pet, such as listening to the melodic song of a beautiful yellow canary rather than wrestling with a rambunctious German shepherd.

Certain stroke patients can't speak, but the unspoken communication between animal and human can be a vital link, and needs no actual words. Certainly, companion animals are capable of helping humans with disabilities from stroke during their daily activities and as part of their rigorous and often long periods of rehabilitation.

PAIN, PAIN, GO AWAY

Chronic pain from cancer and other life-threatening conditions hampers real life for many people, every day, says Dr. Ann Berger, an oncologist in pain and palliative care at the National Institutes of Health. At NIH, doctors are running clinical trials with the most experimental of medicines. But they are also exploring alternative and complementary types of medicine. Holding or simply touching a beloved pet stacks up as one vital cog in the wheel of pain treatment.

"Suffering is only helped with bringing in all the other fields we can," says Dr. Berger. "We need spiritual care people, because even if somebody's not religious, it's always a spiritual care issue. It's always, 'Why me? Why is this happening to me?' You can use art. You can use music. Pet therapy helps some patients. And that's where we get the most work done."

If you're in pain, try a terrier, not a Tylenol! Pets, especially cats and dogs, miraculously zero in when and where we are hurting. They leap lightly with agility when joining us in bed, and in some inexplicable way curl up as a furry bandage to soothe what ails us.

PART THREE

Deepening the Bond

Getting the Most Out of
Your Relationship

EVEN AMONG THOSE OF US who indulge our pets like favorite grandchildren, there is room to optimize intimacy and the Bond. I mistakenly thought the relationship I shared with my pets was already at its peak. But I was soon to discover that my level of intimacy with my own pets was as shallow as a birdbath, when it had the capacity to be as deep as the ocean.

I experienced this rude awakening after I took the same tests I am sharing with you in this section. I felt my lifetime of experience with pets had given me a well-trained eye. My pets were happy and healthy, or so I thought. I was shocked when the Becker Bond-O-Meter test results rated a C minus, not the A plus I was expecting.

To deepen the Bond with your pet, you need to spend time together. One good night kiss from Sirloin and I knew my pets had dismissible, not kissable breath. One look at a growing mat of hair near LLLucky's rump and I knew that he needed regular brushing to have a huggable coat. I knew Scooter craved physical contact, and our cats, Turbo and Tango, had been left to entertain themselves. If your pet has a huggable coat, kissable breath, and enjoys your playtime together as much as you do, you will feel more deeply Bonded.

I looked at my report card, and my spirits sank. The health and well-being of my cherished pets was being compromised by simple ignorance and unconscious actions. I saw that I was guilty of inconsistency. What's more, my pets were paying the price of my hectic schedule by receiving quick pats on their heads, rushed walks, and broken promises of evening playtimes. So I did what any struggling student should: I got tutoring.

I interviewed experts in canine and feline well-being. Then with equal parts skepticism and enthusiasm, I digested this new information and experimented with changing my ways. My goal in this "in-the-trenches" testing was to see if these innovations, some of which I thought were pretty silly, would take our dogs and cats from what most would consider a happy, healthy, full life to canine nirvana and feline ecstasy. By paying closer attention to my dogs and cats, I learned how to rev up their daily rituals to maximize the Bond between us. I also learned how to focus on their true wants and needs. Now I can commend to you the process I went through. Optimizing the Bond is the best gift you can give your pet (and yourself), better than a catnip-filled toy mouse or a juicy piece of steak.

How do you rate your relationship with your pet? And what can you do to get closer to the ideal relationship? In this section, I will provide essential tactics and tools to help you strengthen your Bond.

Quiz Time: Grading Your
People-Pet Bond

TAKE A MOMENT TO COMPLETE the IdealPet™ Program Quizzes. These quick tests are designed to assess how your dog and cat size up when compared to your ideal pet and to help you unleash your pet's own unique genetic potential. The IdealPet™ Program is the pet version of the U.S. Army slogan "Be all you can be."

And remember that you play a major role in the outcome of the IdealPet™ Program. Only by true understanding and clear communication with your pet can you achieve the best possible relationship. Working with Dr. Rolan Tripp, we have developed a new approach to making your dog or cat happier, more playful, and loving.

The IdealPet™ Program isn't intended to focus on your flaws or those of your pet. Rather, it's designed to steer you and your pet closer to achieving your own idea of people-pet nirvana.

IdealDog™ Tests:

Even if you think you already have an ideal dog, take this test anyway to see how your pooch compares. The more "yes" answers you check, the closer you are to experiencing your ideal.

IDEALHOUSEDOG™

Let's see how your dog stacks up as a houseguest. Answer yes or no to describe your dog's household habits and patterns.

1.	Eliminates reliably in designated pet toilet areas	yes	no
2.	Sits when requested under any circumstance	yes	no
3.	Stays off specified furniture unless invited	yes	no
4.	Moves out of your way when asked	yes	no
5.	Ignores trash and chewable items that are off limits	yes	no
6.	Greets new people in a friendly manner on cue	yes	no
7.	Resists rushing out the door, or roaming the neighborhood	yes	no
8.	Goes to a specified location upon request and waits quietly	yes	no
9.	Demonstrates contentment in a crate or when tethered	yes	no
10.	Stays off people and does not jump up to greet them	yes	no
11.	Barks to alert you but does not make excessive, unwanted noise	yes	no
12.	Accepts nail trimming, tooth brushing, and bathing with patience	yes	no
13.	Meets visiting children without showing signs of aggression	yes	no
14.	Comes when called inside the house	yes	no
15.	Displays no interest in household destruction	yes	no

16. Finds car keys, TV remote, or other scent-   yes no
marked item upon request

17. Appears to be close to ideal weight   yes no

18. Shows a glossy, luxurious coat   yes no

19. Does not have bad breath   yes no

    16–19   Graduated magna cum laude from Good Dog U.
    12–15   Spent Mom and Dad's college money wisely
     8–11   I knew he shouldn't have joined that fraternity
 7 or below   Matchbook degree going up in flames

THE IDEALCOMPANIONDOG™

Try this test to see how your dog stacks up as a delightful exercise/ traveling companion.

1. Comes immediately when called while off leash yes no
at a park or beach

2. Stops at every curb and waits for permission to yes no
proceed

3. Meets new dogs without acting aggressive or yes no
unruly

4. Plays nicely with familiar dogs yes no

5. Behaves as a considerate passenger in any vehicle yes no

6. Heels on lead in a crowd yes no

7. Heels off lead in a safe area yes no

8. Eliminates on command, in specified locations yes no

9. Enters and rests quietly in a dog crate when yes no
requested

10. Rests quietly in a down-stay position until yes no
released

11. Acts reliably around children and adults when yes no
out in public

12. Stops barking when given the signal yes no

13. Responds as directed when approached by a stranger   yes   no

14. Accepts body handling and grooming without fear or aggression   yes   no

15. Travels comfortably in a crate, car, bus, or airplane   yes   no

12–15	AAA five-star rating
9–11	We'll keep the light on for you
6–8	A pet hostel is your best shot
5 or below	Can't you read the sign? Pets not welcome!

IDEALTRICKDOG™

How does your dog rate when it comes to mastering a bag of canine tricks? Put your dog through this screen test to see if you have a dog whiz kid.

1. Sit-shake—Sits and offers paw to greet people   yes   no

2. Stand-shake—Stands and offers paw to people   yes   no

3. Roll over—Rolls over and over until cued to stop   yes   no

4. Yes and no—Shakes head "yes" or "no" on cue   yes   no

5. Bang—Plays dead, lying completely still   yes   no

6. Play possum—Lies on back with all four legs up   yes   no

7. Bark—Speaks on command   yes   no

8. Back—Walks backward   yes   no

9. Station—Goes to a mat and lies down   yes   no

10. Fetch—Retrieves any requested item such as a ball, stick, or Frisbee   yes   no

11. Doorbell dash—Runs to a mat when the doorbell rings   yes   no

12. Figure 8—Walks through and around your legs   yes   no

13. Boinga, boinga—Jumps up with all four legs   yes   no
off the ground

14. Take a bow—Bows on command   yes   no

15. Vacuum—Cleans up the spilled food on the   yes   no
floor

12–15	A fur-covered Copperfield
8–11	Lounge act in Vegas
4–7	Good entertainment for a child's birthday party
3 or below	Able to make human family disappear with embarrassment

IDEALSHOWDOG ™

Is your dog ready to wow them at Westminster, or do fabulously at the local 4-H show? See how your dog compares to blue-ribbon performers.

1. Heels on and off lead at various speeds   yes   no

2. Stays in the down position out of owner's   yes   no
sight for up to five minutes

3. Stays in a sit position out of owner's sight for   yes   no
up to two minutes

4. Stays in a stand position out of owner's sight   yes   no
for up to one minute

5. Goes away from owner, drops, then returns to   yes   no
owner on command

6. Performs sit, down, or stand from a distance   yes   no
on command

7. Jumps on or off a table when requested   yes   no

8. Retrieves the specified object and places in   yes   no
owner's hand

9. Discriminates scents, finds object marked by a   yes   no
person's scent

10. Jumps over any safe, reasonable object   yes   no

11. Crawls through a tube when exit is not visible   yes   no

12. Climbs a reasonable obstacle to continue a path   yes   no

13. Jumps through a reasonable hoop   yes   no

14. Registered to compete in American Kennel Club   yes   no
    obedience trials

12–14	Howl-e-wood Superstar—featured in *Dogue* magazine
9–11	Miss Am-hair-ica semifinalist
6–8	Judges found out your mother had fleas
5 or below	You'll get more than "fifteen minutes of shame"

Dogs Think They're Human; Cats Think They're God

Many people consider the cat to be essentially an independent, self-domesticated animal that until very recently was valued primarily for its unparalleled abilities as an exterminator of vermin. Nothing, however, could be farther from the truth. Yes, cats have been known to single-clawedly control vermin populations, and yes, thanks to cats we are spared the second coming of bubonic plague. But even more important than their rodent control value is their status as a living and timeless symbol of hearth and home. What image so conjures up peace, contentment, and security as a sleeping cat or kitten curled up on your favorite chair? And what sound could be more sweetly soothing than a well-modulated purr?

It should come as no surprise that at about the same time that the use of drugs such as Prozac and Zoloft became popular, cats began to overtake dogs as the most popular pet in America. Felines of all colors, shapes, and breeds are nature's finest antistress, draped over-the-counter medicine.

As any veteran cat owner can attest, cats march to their own internal drum. If they feel like a back rub, they jump onto your newspaper guilt-free, just as you've settled down to read it. Count on your cat to walk across your keyboard—or drape across your mouse—if you are frantically aiming for a deadline on a report. Only the strong or the stressed can resist dropping everything to oblige her every need. A cat can bring a smile to your face and a reminder to slow down a little. Shouldn't every office or home have one?

Here's how to make the Bond you share with your cat really purr.

IdealCat™ *Tests*

Is your feline fabulously fine? Again, check "yes" or "no" after each statement. The more "yes" responses, the closer you are to being in the proud company of your ideal cat.

(NB: Dr. Tripp did not include an IdealShowCat™ test as show cats are not required to perform tasks at shows.)

IdealHouseCat™

1.	Runs to greet me when I come home	yes	no
2.	Eagerly seeks gentle handling and petting	yes	no
3.	Likes to curl up on my lap	yes	no
4.	Eliminates only in approved litter locations	yes	no
5.	Comes when called for food	yes	no
6.	Acts friendly and confident when meeting new people	yes	no
7.	Does not destroy household items	yes	no
8.	Accepts food treats politely without grabbing or biting	yes	no
9.	Stays relaxed while being bathed	yes	no
10.	Plays enthusiastically with a variety of toys	yes	no
11.	Keeps off designated counters and furniture	yes	no
12.	Is not overweight	yes	no
13.	Does not have bad breath	yes	no

10–13	My cat is an honor student at Feline High
6–9	My cat is a student athlete who sees C's on each report card
5 or below	My cat has a promising career in the fast-food industry

IDEALCOMPANIONCAT™

Take this test to see how your cat rates as the purr-fect partner for trips around the block or just hanging out together at home.

1. Walks easily on a harness and leash — yes   no
2. Enters a portable kennel when requested — yes   no
3. Remains calm and relaxed while traveling in the portable kennel — yes   no
4. Stays relaxed around friendly children — yes   no
5. Enjoys petting from friendly strangers — yes   no
6. Allows handling and being held by strangers — yes   no
7. Accepts grooming without showing aggression or stress — yes   no

6–7	A Mobile five-star rating
4–5	I'll wear fur proudly on this trip
3 or below	Did you say alley cat?

IDEALTRICKCAT™

How does your cat rate when it comes to doing some "meowi-wow-whee" kind of tricks that will dazzle your friends?

1. Comes when called — yes   no
2. Meows on cue — yes   no
3. Sits and lies down when requested — yes   no
4. Sits and stays for a short time — yes   no
5. Sits up ("begs") — yes   no
6. Jumps up or down from any reasonable location — yes   no
7. "Dances" (up on hind legs) — yes   no
8. Gives a high five on cue — yes   no
9. Rolls over on cue — yes   no
10. Retrieves thrown objects — yes   no

8–10	A star is born!
5–7	You got the meow mojo working, baby!
3–4	Get a new agent
2 or below	Don't call us, we'll call you.

Health Care Checklist

OUR PETS MEAN THE WORLD to us. Just loving them can improve our health, and they need us to help them keep in tiptop shape. Begin each month by running through my twenty-six-point pet home health care checklist. These monthly "checkups" can help nip any problems in the bud, thus protecting your pet from unnecessary pain, expense . . . or worse. A "no" answer to any of these questions is a trigger to immediately call your veterinarian or take your pet in for a "hands-on" checkup.

My Pet:

1. Is acting normal and appears to be in good spirits   yes   no

2. Does not tire easily with moderate exercise   yes   no

3. Does not have seizures or fainting episodes   yes   no

4. Has a normal appetite with no significant weight change   yes   no

5. Does not vomit or regurgitate food   yes   no

6. Has normal-appearing bowel movements (firm, formed, mucus-free)   yes   no

7. Does not drag or scoot around on his bottom   yes   no

8. Has a full, glossy coat with no missing hair, matting, or excessive shedding   yes   no

9. Does not scratch, lick, or chew himself excessively   yes   no

10. Does not have inflamed pink or red skin, dry flakes, odor, and is not greasy   yes   no

11. Is free from fleas, ticks, lice, or mites   yes   no

12. Has a body free of lumps or bumps   yes   no

13. Has ears that are clean and odor-free   yes   no

14. Does not shake his head or paw at his ears   yes   no

15. Has eyes that are clear, bright, and free of discharge   yes   no

16. Has normal hearing and reacts as usual to his home surroundings   yes   no

17. Walks without stiffness, pain, or difficulty   yes   no

18. Has healthy-looking feet and short nails (dew claws, too!)   yes   no

19. Breathes normally without straining or coughing   yes   no

20. Has a normal thirst and drinks the usual amount each day   yes   no

21. Urinates in the usual amounts and frequency and the color is normal   yes   no

22. Has a moist nose that is free from discharge   yes   no

23. Has clean, white teeth free from tartar, plaque, or bad breath   yes   no

24. Has gums that are pink with no redness,   yes   no
    swelling, or bad breath

25. Has no offensive habits (biting, digging,   yes   no
    barking, chewing, spraying)

26. Is housetrained and eliminates on a regular   yes   no
    schedule

Achieving the Ultimate Bond

I HOPE THESE TESTS HAVE heightened your awareness of the many ways you relate to your pets and helped you to uncover even more pathways to gaining the "Ultimate Bond." Feel like you have a better gauge on your pet's levels of health and happiness? Now we're ready to take the plunge deeper into the IdealDog™ or IdealCat™ zone. Let's begin with what I affectionately call the "love loop."

The by-product of loving your pet in a new, more connective way is a Bond that is honed on a hormonal and neurological level. To keep it simple, let's look at what you can incorporate into your pet's daily rituals to become the love master in your pet's life. Our love master recipe includes therapeutic touch, increased interactive play, brushing teeth, grooming, or even preparing an occasional special treat or homemade meal. We will even explore different ways you can talk to your pets.

Finally, we'll learn the importance of pet parenting and how to get back to basics, such as letting dogs be dogs and cats be cats. As successful pet parents, we will begin to understand innate species tendencies, and thereby resist the temptation to transform our pets into little four-legged humans in fur coats.

The Love Loop

Picture three couples, all deeply in love, sitting on a single park bench. Perched on one end is a young couple. He is stroking her hair and she is rubbing the nape of his neck as they stare deeply into each other's eyes. Hormones surge!

On the opposite end of the bench is a mother cradling her infant child, an image that universally broadcasts love and contentment. The baby coos as the mother talks lovingly and caresses her baby's face with the feather-light strokes of her fingertips. These sights, sounds, and touches act as a catalyst for a mixture of powerful instincts in the central nervous systems of each participant.

Sitting in the middle of the bench is an elderly man who repeatedly pets the length of a small dog resting in his lap. The man looks down, catches the sleepy dog's gaze, and tells his friend how much Daddy loves him. Again, for this couple, hormones synergistically surge.

In each of these examples, the intensity and duration of the experience feeds back and forth in a continuous love loop. What is being developed is a close, familiar, affectionate, and loving exchange—intimacy—that results in what could best be described as a total mind-body hormonal spa treatment. Anxiety and tension leave the body. With a love loop, a serene nervous system subconsciously uses the hormonal system to communicate with the immune system for optimum efficiency and incredible physical, emotional, and psychological benefits. Science is finally painting in the numbers of the love loop, creating a physical and emotional masterpiece that we've known to exist for years.

The skin is the body's largest organ, and is the most complex source of sensory input to the brain. It not only reports touch, but also pain, temperature, and pressure. Based on all this input, combined with pre-existing nature and nurture factors, the brain releases endocrine hormones that ultimately control the immune system. A confused, anxious brain sends muddled messages, confounding the immune system. A relaxed, loving brain allows the body and mind to work in natural harmony. This is the mechanism that explains why the love loop has such a healing power.

Rebecca Johnson, Ph.D., RN, of the University of Missouri–Columbia, citing the work of researchers such as her colleague Prof. Johannes Odendaal of South Africa, says that scientists can now recognize the whole physiological chain of events from sensory input to neurohormone release. One love loop example is how touch can help release prolactin, which stimulates social bonding, and oxytocin, which facilitates tactile contact.

Oxytocin receptors are in areas of the brain involved with joyous and affectionate behavior, Rebecca Johnson says. As these feel-good, nurturing, natural biochemicals are released, we should expect the individual—whether it's animal or human—to seek out situations that enable these effects. Pets and people seek pleasure and avoid pain. The beauty of the Bond is that we can do it together.

The image of dogs or cats who lick themselves to heal conjures up a powerful image of how their licking can, in fact, heal us. Each time you pet your dog or cat—and they lick you—take comfort in knowing you are participating in one of the oldest healing rituals known to mankind. Picture my six-foot, two-inch brother Bob having his aching knees and feet sponge bathed by the hyperactive tongue of Buddy, his determined Yorkshire terrier. I have seen the grimace of his pain turn into a grin as the chemical spa treatment took effect.

In the love loop, intimate contact with your pet allows healing powers to flow to and from both of you. *Look, listen, touch,* and *talk* are the keys to the ignition and the fuel of this love loop. You've heard that more is better, and in this case it's true. It's no wonder that extending the time you spend in the love loop, cooing and petting, increases your payback. Chances are, you'll get the cat purring or the dog's tail wagging with delight, causing you to engage more fully, making the pet respond even more positively.

With pets, the process of intimacy seems easy. Society puts so many pressures upon us and places so much emphasis on individuality that in contrast, pets make it possible to love unconditionally and in abundance. Reality says that long after the couple at one end of the bench has moved on to other relationships, and the toddler has grown up to be a recalcitrant teenager, the pet is still going to be in your world and gazing at you with "the look of love." A pet may grow old, but it never grows out of the need to be near you.

Animal Amenities: Huggable Coat, Kissable Breath, Massage, Comfort, Purposeful Play, and Home Cooking

For optimal performance, this love loop requires putting specific strategies into action. In your quest to develop a closer relationship with your pet, I've discovered that some of the best Bond enhancers include huggable coats, kissable breath, therapeutic massages, fun, interactive games, and serving an occasional homemade meal that caters to your cat or dog's taste buds without sacrificing nutrition.

HUGGABLE COAT

A pet will not last on a lap or sleep nose-to-nose with their loved one reeking of cologne de dirty dog. Is your pet's coat so gnarly and smelly that you'd like to unzip it and take it to a Laundro-mutt, if you could? All breeds require some kind of regular grooming. Sirloin, our Labrador retriever, gets a bath every other month. Scooter is professionally groomed once a month, and has a bath at home every other week. Turbo and Tango, the short-haired barn cats, groom themselves. My rule of thumb is the pet should be huggable—if it's not, it needs a bath.

Regular grooming also makes your pet more comfortable and healthier. Imagine what you'd look and feel like if you never washed or brushed your hair. A single mat of hair can contain hundreds of hairs all twisted together. Once the mat gets wet, it shrinks like a wool sweater pulling tighter and tighter, until it becomes painful and irritates the skin underneath. And by the way, do not call, "Come get your bath." Just bring your dog to the grooming site and give them a treat. If the experience is perceived as no fun, the word "come" could become a negative signal and its use for other situations, such as an emergency call to come away from the street, could be diminished.

Boy, do pets have keen senses! When Scooter hears the first drips of water hitting the bottom of the bathtub, the imperceptible creak of the cupboard door that contains the dog shampoo opening, or the sound of the nail trimmers being laid on the counter, she starts slinking off to the deepest, darkest recesses of our house, trying to make herself invisible. The same dog that doesn't hear you when you scream, "Come here!" is able to detect the faint whisper, "I think I'll give Scooter a bath."

Before bathing, feed the dog in the bathtub periodically, and especially a few days before bath time. Keep irresistibly tasty treats handy, and give one during the bath to reward acceptance, but never right after shaking or any attempt to leave the tub. To prepare, put a bath mat or towel in the bottom of the tub (even if it already has no-slip strips in the bottom). For those brave souls who bathe their cats, a small section of window screen will provide something to latch onto. Put a ball of steel wool in the drain to catch hair, plug your pet's ears loosely with cotton (*Don't* forget to take them out!), and put a drop of mineral oil or a little ophthalmic ointment in the eyes to protect them from shampoo.

Take the pet—don't call him to the tub—and douse his body, not his head, with lukewarm water. Keep his head dry until the very last part of the bath. This is important because water dripping off of his face and ears triggers shaking. Use a high-quality pet shampoo and conditioner that is pH-balanced for pets, not people; or a therapeutic shampoo recommended by your veterinarian. Work up a good lather on the body and then work down the neck and back.

To prevent your pet from shaking dry and bathing you while lathering, drape a large towel over his back while you work on the rest of the body. This towel keeps the pet warm and 90 percent of the water in the towel, and not on you or in the room if they shake. If you like a high-gloss coat, apply a veterinarian-approved coat conditioner or cream rinse to make his coat smoother and easier to brush. Conditioners make grooming easier both this time, and next. Rinse well! Blot his coat with a terry towel to remove moisture or use a hairdryer, pointing the nozzle at a section of wet hair as you simultaneously brush. If the weather is cold, keep your pet inside until dry.

No matter what you do for grooming on the outside of your dog, you need to feed its coat from "the inside out" with veterinary-recommended foods that are nutrient-rich and formulated to give your pet healthy skin, a shiny, luxurious coat, and vigor. Veterinarians and groomers can tell from a mile away which pets are fed premium foods, as their coats announce it like a neon sign.

Most pets love to be brushed, especially if started early in life. Think of what it feels like to have someone rhythmically brush your hair or massage your scalp during shampooing. Aaaaah. Just imagining it is therapeutic. Because pets' coats differ so much, what you use for short-haired Sirloin wouldn't work very well on long-haired LLLucky. And cats have sensitive skin, so they need a softer brush than dogs do.

KISSABLE BREATH

As a veterinarian, I know a broken tooth is a bacterial superhighway leading directly to the bloodstream. I know how incredibly bioactive periodontal disease is, and that with every bite, a pet with "Billy Bob" teeth is pumping bacteria directly into the bloodstream. This bacteria in the bloodstream, or bacteremia, is an invisible killer that does major long-term damage to the liver, kidneys, and the heart. I also know that the term "hurts like a toothache" lives up to its billing, and that at times my pet's breath smelled like limburger cheese on the Fourth of July.

If I knew my negligence was slowly poisoning my pets, causing them discomfort, and keeping us at arm's length, why wasn't I doing something about it? The fact is that 85 percent of pets over three years of age have dental disease. When people say, "My pet's mouth doesn't look that bad," veterinary dentist Dr. Tom Mulligan says in retort, "How would you like *your* mouth to look that way?"

Not only can doggie breath be greatly reduced or even eliminated with frequent brushing and regular professional care, brushing your pet's teeth can easily add two years to its life, says veterinary dentist Dr. Jan Bellows. With that mandate, I started with our dogs.

I began slowly, with safety being uppermost in my mind. Nobody wants to be bitten, even accidentally. I started out rubbing my pets' faces, then spent time gently lifting up their lips and touching their teeth with my fingers. Then I progressed to rubbing the toothbrush on the sides of their faces and touching their toothbrushes dipped in tuna juice on the sides of the teeth. So far so good.

These aren't Crest pets. Today, pet toothpaste comes in so many lip-smacking flavors—including beef, poultry, fish, and mint—that few pets will turn up their noses at it. Don't use toothpastes designed for humans because they are laden with detergents and are designed for the sequence of brush, spit, and rinse. With pets, what goes in the mouth goes down the hatch, so human toothpaste can cause stomach upsets. I used CET malt-flavored toothpaste, and all the dogs so loved the taste they'd eat it out of the tube like Cheez Whiz if I'd let them. I have some special doggie toothbrushes for the big dogs, and use bristled finger cots for Scooter.

Day by day, my pets became used to the slow, circular motions of the toothbrush waltzing across their teeth, and began to appreciate the time I was spending with them. After a few weeks, rather than Scooter,

Sirloin, and LLLucky fighting my attempts to brush their teeth, they were fighting one another to be first in line. Even though over a period of months they got close to kissable breath, the sight of them wolfing down some horse manure at the corral left me satisfied with a peck on the cheek. But their pearly whites sure look good in family pictures now.

Pets are like humans. If you brushed your own teeth once a week, what would they look like? Ideally, brush your pet's teeth every day, but even if you do it three to four times a week, your veterinarian will give you a gold star and your pet will purr or wag its tail in appreciation. I still haven't got up enough guts to try to brush the teeth of the cats, Turbo and Tango.

MASSAGE

No need to contract out for your pet's personal masseuse. With no experience required, you can fill this bill. Don't underestimate the therapeutic powers of a purposeful touch. Begin slowly. Watch your pet to learn their favorite spots and types of touches. Experiment with grooming tools in addition to the fabulous five-finger method. Learning to massage your pet will definitely strengthen the Bond you share, medical benefits included. And what an investment in a long future together!

To help with time management, consider picking a favorite television program to watch while you begin your first few sessions during commercial breaks. Once the routine is established, pick a time when the television is off and you can give full attention to your pet. Set aside five or ten minutes every day or so, when both of you are calm and free from distractions.

Tell your pet "sweet nothings" in a soothing tone. Apply gentle pressure with your curved hand, with long flowing strokes from head to rump. Use the pads of your thumbs to apply gentle pressure and massage specific points around the eyes, ears, skull, and spine. Allow your fingertips (not your fingernails) to glide, press, tickle, knead, and move all over your pet's body. Pay particular attention to the areas your pet enjoys the most. Don't press too deeply on bony prominences but do feel for areas of muscle tension or where the skin feels hotter. Concentrate on those areas.

During the massage, feel for lumps and scabs; look for fleas or ticks. Most important, tune into your pet's response and learn their feedback signs. If your pet melts into your arms, purrs, pushes up against your hands, becomes a limp rag of relaxation, or rolls around you in utter delight, you'll know you are making the love connection in a big way. If your pet starts to resist, wiggle, or flee, try to do something else you know your pet likes, or promptly end the session.

Dr. Robin Downing, a multi-award–winning veterinarian in Windsor, Colorado, wants her clients to have such a strong physical and emotional relationship with their pets that they can touch them from the tip of their noses to the tips of their tails without the pets objecting. Routine touch builds intimacy and trust with our pets. Pet massages feel good to give and to get. We gain familiarity with every curve and bump on our pet's bodies. Our intuition begins to tell us when something is wrong and needs to be seen by a veterinarian.

Scooter is living proof of the benefits of routine massage. In my search for a way to relieve Scooter's arthritis pain, I spoke with two integrative medicine specialists at Colorado State University College of Veterinary Medicine, Dr. Brenda McClelland and Dr. Narda Robinson. Both experts spent a long time trying to convince me that I should give Scooter frequent massages.

They instructed me to take my right hand and use it to explore every fold of Scooter's ample body, searching for the soreness, taut muscles, and temperature differences that would betray the arthritic pain hidden deep within. I didn't believe them, I confess, but in the spirit of exploration and experimentation that motivated all of these changes, I gave it a try. Like a golfer who hits the perfect swing or a chef who creates a prize-winning recipe, I knew, via Scooter's direct feedback, when my bodywork was hitting her in all the right places in just the right amounts. She started standing on her tippytoes, pushing her body into my hands, with eyes half-closed, panting with desire. She was exhibiting so much pleasure that I felt I should look around to make sure nobody was watching!

Like a harried worker at an airport baggage claim office getting a shoulder and neck massage from a coworker, Scooter grew to love the backrubs and continues to get her thrice-daily dose of the magic, vibrating fingers. Whereas in the past she used to stand parallel to my office chair for a fleeting pat on the head as I worked at my computer, she now backs up to my chair slowly (I imagine her making the sound of a truck that's backing up!) for some serious lingering. I grew to love giving her comfort, and vice versa, as she loved to repay my labor of love in the best way she knew how—giving my face a sponge bath with her raspy tongue.

COMFORT

For Sirloin, we wanted to make his world more comfortable. Having torn the pad out of his Igloo dog house and chewed it into confetti, he'd been sleeping out on the gravel or in the grass with a tattered security blanket he'd been dragging around, Linus-like, for years. When winter was over, we found it frozen into the snow. We rescued it, cleaned it, and put it away to serve as his summer picnic blanket. Then we upgraded him to a big cedar-filled flannel pillow so that when he went into his dog house at night it was like nestling into the most incredible comforter at a country inn.

Three-legged LLLucky likes to collapse onto the ground with a thud and expose his underbelly for some slow stroking. Besides his conveyor-belt tongue spilling out of his mouth in delight, he keeps asking for more by reaching out to touch me with the invisible paw that he thinks is still attached to the stump of a leg that revolves slowly underneath the skin high on his rib cage. As you can see, each dog in our household now demands what we believe are well-deserved prescriptions for routine pampering, which I am only too happy to administer to them.

PURPOSEFUL PLAY

Does your pet bring into your life an extraordinary element of fun, frivolity, and joy? I believe that daily play is better for us in the short term and long run than a once-a-day multiple vitamin. We know that laughter is the best medicine. And what makes laughter? Playtime! From play, we learn, breathe more deeply, let go of stress, connect with others, and live life fully. The same is true for our pets.

When we pull into the driveway at our home, Sirloin and LLLucky reliably break into play. My dogs have the right idea about life. Play is their top priority, even gaining top billing over mealtimes, which are a close second. We humans may not want to make mealtimes so high on our list, but we would be wise to mimic the frivolity and fun our pets so willingly insert into any moment of the day. To be happy, healthy, and well-adjusted, dogs not only love to play, but play to build love.

Who says what's good for our pets is not good for us? So the next time your dog brings you a favorite toy, or the cat is racing around the house with the turbo kicked in, think twice before turning away to finish whatever it is you are doing. There is always room to fit playtime into the smallest moment.

Despite the adage, you *can* teach an old dog new tricks—and refresh his memory on doggie manners in a fun, engaging way. If done right, your dog will see training sessions as a form of playtime. To get your older dog back on track, learn to say "yes" to positive reinforcement and "no" to negative forms of punishments.

Let's say you have an eighty-pound dog that insists on bowling you over with enthusiasm each time you come home from a hectic workday. Protect your body, and your nylons, by training your dog to become your household's official door greeter by sitting automatically whenever someone enters through the front door. Teach him by giving him small treats and plenty of praise each time he sits when you ask him. Only reward his achievements; ignore his mistakes. In time, your dog will learn of the delicious payoff awaiting him if he "sits pretty" instead of rushing the door like a rhino.

Another fun game to play with your dog is "scavenger hunt." Save a portion of your dog's dinner and sharpen his hunting skills. Teach your dog to "find the treat" each night before his meal. Most dogs love to be assigned jobs. Begin this game by first teaching your dog to sit and stay on cue. Then "hide" a treat in plain sight. After your dog waits for a few seconds, say, "Find the treat" and praise him as he gobbles up this found treasure. As your dog gets the hang of this game, start putting treats in less visible places, such as behind a dining room chair, under the coffee table, on the top stair or in the corner of the living room. Remember how many and where you hid the treats, to keep score on how well your dog performed.

CAT TRICK TRAINING 101

When it comes to mastering tricks or commands, dogs don't have a monopoly. As famed big cat circus trainer Gunther Gebel-Williams said, there was just one animal who was pretty close to untrainable, the house

cat. "They do as they please," he said. Some cats do like to learn, however, and will ham it up. The simple secret to cat trick training? Be
consistent, caring, and patient. Keep training sessions short and fun, not
must-do chores.

Will your cat become the next Morris or land a role on the sequel
to the movie *Cats and Dogs*? Probably not. But if you spend time training
your cat in a positive way, you will stimulate his or her mind,
strengthen his or her self-confidence, and build the Bond. In the process,
you will also hone your cat's social skills, bolster the level of trust between you, and encourage your cat to want to seek you out and spend
time with you. In time your cat may even act more like a dog. Bite my
tongue!

Here are two classic dog tricks that you can teach your talented
tabby.

SIT UP, KITTY

Timing is everything when it comes to trick training with cats. Select
a time when your cat is hungry and in a calm, peaceful mood. When
your cat is sitting pretty, approach slowly. Hold a treat an inch or so
over your cat's head. Say sweetly, "Sit up." If your cat tries to swat at
the treat or stands up, don't give her the treat. Instead, wait for your
cat to sit again. Then repeat the "sit up" cue. Give her the treat the second
she sits up and balances her weight on her hind feet. Praise her, saying,
"Good kitty" in a soothing but sincere voice. Repeat this a few times
daily to build understanding of this game. And, when selecting a treat,
always make it an irresistible one—not an everyday treat. You will have
more success!

SHAKE HANDS

Got a friendly cat that likes to greet visitors at the door? Accelerate
your cat's ambassador-like tendencies by teaching her how to shake
hands. Start with your cat positioned in front of you. Touch her front
right paw with a small food treat and say, "Shake." The second she lifts
her paw, gently put your hand under it for a moment, heap on the
praise, and give the treat. In time, you will be able to extend this action
to gently shaking hands. Repeat these steps in sequence four or five

times. Stop the lesson once your cat delivers a couple paw shakes or becomes bored and heads to her cat bed.

HOME COOKING

At least once a week, open up the pantry door and become your pet's personal chef by preparing a homemade meal or tasty treat.

Consult with your veterinarian for recipes that will be meow-va-lous for your cat and bark-a-licious for your dog, and won't cause them any harm. I have stumbled upon a couple tasty treats for Sirloin, my lovable Lab. Occasionally, I soak his hard hollow chew toy (KONG toy) in a meaty broth, or wipe peanut butter or cream cheese inside of it and serve it to him as an appetizer before he gets his regular dog food. It's a dog's version of eating dessert first. Sirloin happily licks and gnaws on this former "rubber yucky" that now tastes great. For a summertime treat for all the dogs, we make frozen cherry or grape Kool-Aid pops in the shape of dog bones. It's a surefire way to make "hot dogs" cool.

We give the cats organic catnip to turn their turbochargers on and keep trying dozens of new cat treats in a quest to find "the" irresistible cat treat that's proving to be as elusive to find as the Holy Grail. Turbo and Tango's main treat is just keeping their food bowl full. Many cats have a problem with territorialism when food is scarce and can become more aggressive. As their veterinarian and purveyor of the can opener, I made an executive decision to let Turbo and Tango be a little fatter but happier. About once a week, Teresa will whip up something special for the kitties when she's cooking chicken or tuna for her salad. When we take it to the barn, their eyes light up like gemstones in a jewelry store display case.

But don't expect too much. Even though pets may have heaps of gourmet food served up in a personalized, designer dog bowl, their instincts might tell them not to overeat, or to eat something rotten. I once caught Sirloin happily munching away on a rotting skunk carcass. Bone appetite!

Aim for Achieving the Bond—Not Bondage

Dogs are very social. Whenever Scooter goes outside the house—to do her business, to get a whiff of fresh air, or chase a chipmunk that ran by an hour ago—and then returns, Sirloin and LLLucky run over to greet her with effusive licks on her mouth and muzzle.

Being social animals, dogs love to keep in touch with their buddies from a distance even when they can't check their pee-mail, moon their friends, or observe visual cues. As a pet parent knows, they do this by throwing their voice around the neighborhood in the canine version of a conference call. Every bark, howl, yip, whine, whimper, or change in pitch is perfectly understood by every dog that hears it. Giant Great Danes speak the same language as tiny Chihuahuas. Various yips, howls, and bellows convey happiness, hurt, fear, loneliness, warnings, even just "Hey, can anybody hear me? Hello? I'm lone, lone, lone, loooooooonley!"

In your dogged pursuit to create an earthly pet paradise, I caution you to not go overboard in your efforts to give your pets everything humanly possible. We're all guilty of excessively heaping human qual-ities and conditions on to our dogs or cats from time to time. We also need to let dogs be dogs and cats be cats. Do not make your pet forsake its true self in order to fit into your rigid mold of ideal human traits or intimacy.

The dulling of the senses of a herding dog who has nothing to herd or a hunting cat who has a window view of prey just out of reach should concern us more than it does. Not being able to fulfill their basic biological and social nature jeopardizes their good health, happiness, and longevity. Many years ago we figured out that animals in a zoo, locked in cages with no stimulation, became frustrated, bored, self-destructive, unhealthy, and unhappy. Pets that are not given appropriate stimula-tion, or worse yet locked in a dog pen or chained up all day, are undergoing the equivalent frustration of solitary confinement.

To really grasp what happens under these circumstances, imagine you're watching a 3-D movie and you're asked to take your glasses off. Then the sound is turned down lower and lower and the colors are muted until the screen becomes only shades of gray. The sounds are there but distant; the same image is still playing in front of you and you can see it, but you can't experience it like before.

That's why we play games of chase with Scooter; let Sirloin hunt and retrieve hidden tennis balls; and play chase and toy games with Turbo and Tango, to hone their hunting reflexes without any lives being taken. We take our horses out of the corral and deep into the mountains where we find a meadow so they can gallop, dispensing energy at maximum horsepower.

As much as pets and people are alike, we're also different. As a friend told me, "Deep in the computer code of a cat and dog are things just waiting to come out with the right sequence of keystrokes." Every time I see a wounded bird fall from hitting the window and Sirloin chase it down before we can save it, Scooter chasing a chipmunk, or Turbo and Tango stalking a grasshopper, I realize that no amount of socialization, behavioral training, human companionship, or reason can override the dog or cat's genetic makeup. Those complex behaviors have been passed down from ancestors and seared into their brains over the millennia. It's within this deeply imprinted genetic code that you must work with your pet to find and fuel behaviors that are desirable in today's modern household.

Instead of trying to rubber-stamp a preferred personality on a pet, foster your pet's unique personality, unshackled by your whims and wants. If you allow your pet to express its natural behaviors, then you, too, will reach the pinnacle of pet-people perfection: the Bond.

WE'RE HOT-WIRED FOR THE BOND

Most of us have felt times when the Bond was nearly perfect. Call it a magical experience, the zone, a call of nature. Rather than trying to overinterpret or second-guess what happened, we should just recognize it for what it is—living proof of the powerful connectedness between mankind and the rest of the animal kingdom—and take steps to make it happen more often.

I once watched my son, Lex, stalking across the grass toward sleeping Sirloin. Objectively, Sirloin is a meat-eating predator weighing about eighty pounds. His gaping mouth opened, revealing curved fangs specifically designed to tear the flesh of prey. As I watched, eleven-year-old Lex decided to mimic some World Championship Wrestling moves he just saw on television and did a full body slam on Sirloin. As Lex landed, Sirloin's lungs let out an explosive blast of air and he awakened from a dream to face a doggie nightmare: I'm under attack!

What did he do? He licked Lex's face and crouched down on his front legs in a play pose ready to take as much abuse as Lex could hand out. Hey, this isn't an attack. It's play! A smile and a wagging tail, laughter and an explosive run by, petting met with licking. A scene repeated in backyards and parks across the world between pets and people. It seems odd when you consider that such a superbly built, intelligent predator would be willing to be used and abused for the sake of play with a weaker and completely different species. If aliens were to land and examine the scene in my yard, unfamiliar with the Bond that has formed between humankind and dogs, they might think humans crazy to engage in hand-to-hand contact or even play with something descended from the wolf, the most feared terminator in its ecosystem.

The mystery of the Bond is that we aren't in even more awe and admiration of it than we are. Of the more than 4,000 species of mammals on this earth, only a few dozen have become domesticated and only two have broken down the doors of our hearts and homes en masse. Demographics show that about six out of ten U.S. households have pets, whereas only three out of ten have children. As Baby Boomers like myself continue to age, our waistlines might be expanding and our hairlines contracting, but our hearts are still in the right place. As nests empty, pets will take on even greater importance as our Bond to life.

Pets are like us and yet other than us. In our symbiosis, we've found that pets are often more humane than humans reflecting the kindest, best impulses of humanity. Pets don't lie or cheat, they have to-die-for loyalty, and then love unconditionally. While these attributes are representative of the rank and file of the pet world, the same can be said for too few humans.

Through our pets, we have a practical, trusted, routine way to relate to nature, to break out of the shackles of mankind and its creations. This relationship, this special affection connection, the Bond, gives us an unparalleled sense of unity with nature; it tells us that we aren't above it, but part of it. Our dogs and cats represent an intimate and enduring look at another mammalian mind and spirit and serve as a thread connecting us back to the expanse of nature. Embedded in this Bond to life is simple, surefire, healing power.

Pets are totems of the values we hold dear and a conduit to our historic connections between humans and nature. They help cultivate the awareness that we are not alone in this world, but united to all living things. They take us outside of ourselves and reacquaint us with the world we live in. Our need for each other, which is part spiritual, part visceral, helps keep us happy and healthy.

Resources

Delta Society®

Delta Society's mission is to improve human health through service and therapy animals. Through their National Service Dog Center™, they provide information to people with service dogs, helping them to become self-advocates and to exercise their rights to access public places under the Americans with Disabilities Act (ADA). Delta Pet Partners® volunteers visit hospitals or hospices with their animals to provide comfort to people in need (known as animal-assisted activity programs).

289 Perimeter Road East
Renton, WA 98055
(425) 226-7357
www.deltasociety.org

Morris Animal Foundation

Morris Animal Foundation is a fifty-three-year-old nonprofit organization that improves the health and well-being of companion animals and wildlife by funding humane health studies and disseminating information about these studies. One hundred percent of annual, unrestricted donations supports animal health studies, not the cost of administration or fund-raising.

45 Inverness Drive East
Englewood, CO 80112
(800) 243-2345
www.morrisanimalfoundation.org

American Animal Hospital Association (AAHA)

Established in 1933, AAHA is an international organization of more than 22,000 veterinary care providers who treat companion animals. Through its hospital evaluation program, AAHA offers accreditation to veterinary practices throughout the United States and Canada that adhere to the association's high standards of excellence. AAHA standards are recognized around the world as the benchmark for quality care in veterinary medicine. For a referral to an AAHA-accredited hospital, simply contact AAHA.

P.O. Box 150899
Denver, CO 80215
(800) 883-6301
www.healthypet.com

American Veterinary Medical Association (AVMA)

Established in 1863, the AVMA and its more than 60,000 members recognize the importance of the human-animal Bond and the veterinarian's role in preserving, protecting, and strengthening relationships between people and animals. AVMA members contribute to the well-being of animals and people through work in clinical practice, public health, regulatory agencies, uniformed services, and research.

1931 North Meacham Road, Suite 100
Schaumburg, IL 60173
(847) 925-8070
www.avma.org

American Humane Association (AHA)

Since 1877, the AHA has been the only national organization serving as an umbrella for member animal shelters. The AHA's national programs include advocacy to improve welfare of pets; promoting adoptions and curbing pet overpopulation; animal shelter support; disaster relief; legislative initiatives; and a child protection division.

63 Inverness Drive East
Englewood, CO 80112
(800) 227-4645
www.americanhumane.org

American Society for the Prevention of Cruelty to Animals (ASPCA)

Founded in 1866, the ASPCA aims to prevent cruelty and alleviate the pain, fear, and suffering of animals by providing local and national programs that assist thousands of animals nationwide. The ASPCA's national programs include the animal poison control center; humane education; companion animal services; and the national shelter outreach program.

424 E. 92nd Street
New York, NY 10128
(212) 876-7700
www.aspca.org

Humane Society of the United States (HSUS)

The Humane Society of the United States, the nation's largest animal protection organization, supports shelters and pet owners in building and enhancing the human-companion animal Bond through its Pets for Life™ campaign. Pets for Life provides solutions—to behavior issues, restrictions in rental housing, and the concerns of allergic, pregnant, or immunocompromised individuals—and promotes animal health care to end the relinquishment, abandonment, and euthanasia of healthy dogs and cats.

2100 L Street, NW
Washington, DC 20037
(202) 452-1100
www.hsus.org

American Kennel Club Headquarters (AKC)

The American Kennel Club, founded in 1884, is one of the nation's oldest sports-governing organizations. It maintains the largest registry of purebred dogs in the world, is responsible for overseeing the governance of the sport of purebred dogs, and keeps records of competitive results. The AKC Canine Health Foundation funds canine health research with a primary focus on genetics. The AKC Companion Animal Recovery is a worldwide twenty-four-hour-a-day pet identification and recovery service for all types of pets.

260 Madison Avenue
New York, NY 10016
(919) 233-9767
www.akc.org

American Association of Pet Dog Trainers (APDT)

APDT is a professional organization of individual trainers who are committed to becoming better trainers through education. The APDT offers individual pet dog trainers a respected and concerted voice in the dog world. It promotes professional trainers to the veterinary profession and increases public awareness of dog-friendly training techniques.

17000 Commerce Parkway, Suite C
Mt. Laurel, NJ 08054
(800) PET-DOGS; Fax: (856) 439-0525
www.apdt.com

Animal Behavior Network (ABN)

The Animal Behavior Network is a resource for anyone interested in learning more about the behavior of pets. The network includes veterinary hospitals, trainers, and consultants. Through ABN it is possible to take an online course, download a behavior topic, or schedule a telephone consultation with a veterinary behavior consultant.

15340 Pastrana Drive
La Mirada, CA 90638
(714) 523-9425
www.AnimalBehavior.net

Bibliography

Anderson, Robert K., Hart, Benjamin L., and Hart, Lynette A., eds. *The Pet Connection*. Minneapolis, Minn.: University of Minnesota Press, 1984.

Beck, Alan, and Katcher, Aaron. *Between Pets and People: The Importance of Animal Companionship*. West Lafayette, Ind.: Purdue University Press, 1996.

Benson, Herbert. *The Relaxation Response*. New York: Avon Books, Inc., 2000.

Bustad, Leo K. *Compassion: Our Last Great Hope*. Renton, Wash.: Delta Society, 1996.

Cobb, Edith. *The Ecology of Imagination in Childhood*. Dallas, Tex.: Spring Publications, Inc., 1997.

Darwin, Charles. *The Expression of Emotions in Man and Animals*. Chicago, Ill.: The University of Chicago Press, 1965.

Diamond, Jared. *The Third Chimpanzee: The Evolution and Future of the Human Animal*. New York: HarperPerennial, 1993.

Dossy, Larry. *Healing Words: The Power of Prayer and the Practice of Medicine*. New York: HarperPaperbacks, 1997.

Fine, Aubrey. *The Handbook on Animal Assisted Therapy: Theoretical Foundations and Guidelines for Practice*. San Diego, Calif.: Academic Press, 2000.

Friedman, Meyer, and Rosenman, Ray H. *Type A Behavior and Your Heart*. New York: Alfred A. Knopf, Inc., 1974.

Goleman, Daniel. *Emotional Intelligence*. New York: Bantam Books, 1995.

Hart, Benjamin, and Hart, Lynette. *The Perfect Puppy: How to Choose Your Dog by Its Behavior*. New York: W. H. Freeman and Company, 1988.

Katz, Mark. *On Playing a Poor Hand Well: Insights from the Lives of Those Who Have Overcome Childhood Risks and Adversities*. New York: W. W. Norton & Company, 1997.

Knapp, Caroline. *Pack of Two: The Intricate Bond Between People and Dogs.* New York: Random House, 1998.

Kowalski, Gary. *The Souls of Animals.* Walpole, N.H.: Stillpoint Publishing Inc., 1999.

Levinson, Boris. *Pet-Oriented Child Psychotherapy*, 2nd ed. Springfield, Ill.: Charles C. Thomas Publisher, Ltd., 1997.

Lynch, James J. *A Cry Unheard: New Insights into the Medical Consequences of Loneliness.* Baltimore, Md.: Bancroft Press, 2000.

Mack, Arien, ed. *Humans and Other Animals.* Columbus, Ohio: Ohio State University Press, 1999.

Marshall Thomas, Elisabeth. *The Social Lives of Dogs: The Grace of Canine Company.* New York: Simon & Schuster, 2000.

McElroy, Susan Chernak. *Animals as Guides for the Soul: Stories of Life-Changing Encounters.* New York: Ballantine Wellspring, 1998.

McLoughlin, John C. *The Canine Clan: A New Look at Man's Best Friend.* New York: The Viking Press, 1983.

Melson, Gail. *Why the Wild Things Are: Animals in the Lives of Children.* Cambridge, Mass.: Harvard University Press, 2001.

Montagu, Ashley. *Touching: The Human Significance of the Skin.* New York: Harper & Row, 1986.

Moussaieff Masson, Jeffrey. *When Elephants Weep: The Emotional Lives of Animals.* New York: Dell Publishing, 1995.

Newbry, Jonica. *The Pact for Survival: Humans and Their Animal Companions.* Sydney, Australia: ABC Books, 1997.

Pert, Candace B. *Molecules of Emotion: The Science behind Mind-Body Medicine.* New York: Touchstone, 1997.

Pipher, Mary. *Reviving Ophelia: Saving the Selves of Adolescent Girls.* New York: Ballantine Books, 1994.

Randour, Mary Lou. *Animal Grace: Entering a Spiritual Relationship with Our Fellow Creatures.* Novato, Calif.: New World Library, 2000.

Robinson, I. *The Waltham Book of Human-Animal Interactions: Benefits and Responsibilities.* London: Pergamon Open Learning, 1995.

Scott, John Paul, and Fuller, John L. *Genetics and the Social Behavior of the Dog.* Chicago, Ill.: The University of Chicago Press, 1965.

Serpell, James. *In the Company of Animals: A Study of Human-Animal Relationships.* Cambridge: Cambridge University Press, 1986.

Shepard, Paul. *The Others: How Animals Made Us Human.* Washington, D.C.: Island Press, 1997.

———. *Thinking Animals: Animals and the Development of Human Intelligence*. Athens, Ga.: University of Georgia Press, 1998.

Sinatra, Stephen T. *Heartbreak and Heart Disease, A Mind/Body Prescription for Healing the Heart*. New Canaan, Conn.: Keats Publishing, 1999.

Tellington-Jones, Linda, with Taylor, Sybil. *The Tellington TTouch: A Revolutionary Natural Method to Train and Care for Your Favorite Animal*. New York: Penguin Books, 1993.

Thomas, William H. *Life Worth Living: How Someone You Love Can Still Enjoy Life in a Nursing Home. The Eden Alternative in Action*. Acton, Mass.: VanderWyk & Burnham, 1996.

Wiebers, D. *Stroke-Free for Life: The Complete Guide to Stroke Prevention and Treatment*. New York: HarperCollins, 2001.

Wilson, Cindy C., and Turner, Dennis C. *Companion Animals in Human Health*. Thousand Oaks, Calif.: Sage Publications, 1997.

Wilson, Edward O. *Biophilia: The Human Bond with Other Species*. Cambridge, Mass.: Harvard University Press, 1984.

Wilson, Edward O., and Kellert, Stephen R., eds. *The Biophilia Hypothesis*. Washington, D.C.: Island Press, 1993.

Winnicott, D. W. *Playing and Reality*. New York: Routledge, 1989.

Zink, M. Christine. *Peak Performance: Coaching the Canine Athlete*. Lutherville, Md.: Canine Sports Productions, 1997.

Scientific Studies

Allen, K. M., and Blascovich, J. The value of service dogs for people with severe ambulatory disabilities: a randomized controlled trial. *Journal of the American Medical Association* 275, no. 13 (1996): 1001–1006.

Allen, K. M., Blascovich, J., Tomaka, J., Kelsey, R. M. Presence of human friends and pet dogs as moderators of autonomic responses to stress in women. *Journal of Personality and Social Psychology* 61 (1991): 582–589.

Anderson, W., Reid, P., and Jennings, G. L. Pet ownership, and risk factors for cardiovascular disease. *Medical Journal of Australia* 157 (1992): 298–301.

Baker, L. Cerebral palsy and therapeutic riding. *NARHA Strides Magazine* 1 (1995): 1.

Batson, K., McCabe, B., Baun, M. M., and Wilson, C. The effect of a therapy dog on socialization and physiological indicators of stress in persons diagnosed with Alzheimer's disease. In C. Wilson and D. Turner, eds., *Companion Animals in Human Health*. Thousand Oaks, Calif.: Sage Publications, 1998, pp. 203–215.

Baun, M. M., Bergstrom, N., Langston, N., and Thoma, L. Physiological effects of human/companion animal bonding. *Nursing Research* 33 (1984): 126–129.

Baun, M. M., and McCabe, B. The role animals play in enhancing quality of life for the elderly. In A. Fine, ed., *The Handbook on Animal Assisted Therapy*. San Diego, Calif.: Academic Press, 2000, pp. 237–251.

Baun, M. M., Oetting, K., and Bergstrom, N. Health benefits of companion animals in relation to physiologic indices of relaxation. *Holistic Nursing Practice* 5 (1991): 16–23.

Beck, A. M. "Animal Contact and the Older Person: Companionship, Health and the Quality of Life." Paper delivered to the May 1996 AARP Biennial Convention.

———. The use of animals to benefit humans: Animal Assisted Therapy. In A. Fine, ed., *The Handbook on Animal Assisted Therapy*. San Diego, Calif.: Academic Press, 2000, pp. 21–40.

Beck, A. M., and Katcher, A. H. A new look at pet-facilitated therapy. *Journal of the American Veterinary Medical Association* 184 (1984): 414–421.

Bodmer, N. M. Impact of pet ownership on the well-being of adolescents with few familial resources. In C. Wilson and D. Turner, eds., *Companion Animals in Human Health*. Thousand Oaks, Calif.: Sage Publications, 1998, pp. 237–247.

Booth, F., Gordon, S. E., Carlson, C. J., and Hamilton, M. Waging war on modern chronic diseases: Primary prevention through exercise biology. *Journal of Applied Physiology* 88 (2000) 774–87.

Brickel, C. M. Depression in the nursing home: A study using pet-facilitated psychotherapy. In R. Anderson, B. Hart, and L. Hart, eds., *The Pet Connection*. Minneapolis, Minn.: University of Minnesota Press, 1984, pp. 407–415.

Brooks, Suz. "Working with Animals in a Healing Context." Unpublished paper based on her work as a therapist at Green Chimneys.

Bryant, B. K. The neighborhood walk: Sources of support in middle childhood. *Monographs of the Society for Research in Child Development* 50, no. 109 (1985): 3–38.

———. "The Relevance of Pets and Neighborhood Animals to the Social-Emotional Functioning and Development of School-Age Children." Final report to the Delta Society, Renton, Wash., 1987.

————. The richness of child-pet relationships: A consideration of both benefits and cost of pets to children. *Anthrozoos* 3 (1990): 253–261.

Centers for Disease Control, National Institute for Diabetes and Digestive and Kidney Diseases, division of National Institutes of Health website statistics on obesity, diabetes and sedentary lifestyle: http://www.niddk.nih.gove/health/nutrit/pubs/statobes.htm#cost.

Chen, M., Daly, M., Williams, N., Williams, S., Williams, C., and Williams, G. Non-invasive detection of hypoglycemia using a novel, fully biocompatible and patient friendly alarm system. *British Medical Journal* 321 (2000): 1565–1566.

Churchill, M., Safaoui, J., McCabe, B., and Baun, M. Using a therapy dog to alleviate the agitation and desocialization of people with Alzheimer's disease. *Journal of Psychiatric Nursing* 37, no. 4 (1999): 16–22.

Collis, G. M., and McNicholas, J. A theoretical basis for health benefits of pet ownership: Attachment versus psychological support. In C. Wilson and D. Turner, eds., *Companion Animals in Human Health.* Thousand Oaks, Calif.: Sage Publications, 1998, pp. 105–122.

Connel, C. M., and Lago, D. J. Favorable attitudes toward pets and happiness among the elderly. In R. Anderson, B. Hart, and L. Hart, eds., *The Pet Connection* Minneapolis, Minn.: University of Minnesota Press, 1984, pp. 241–250.

Craig, F. W., Lynch, J. J., and Qaurtner, J. L. The perception of available social support is related to reduced cardiovascular reactivity in Phase II cardiac rehabilitation patients. *Inter Physiol Behav Sci* 35, no. 4 (Oct.–Dec. 2000): 272–283.

Dismuke, R. Rehabilitative horseback riding for children with language disorders. In R. Anderson, B. Hart, and L. Hart, eds., *The Pet Connection.* Minneapolis, Minn.: University of Minnesota Press, 1984, pp. 131–140.

Doody, R. S., Stevens, J. C., Beck, C., Dubinsky, R. M., Kaye, J. A., Gwyther, L., Mohs, R. C., Thal, L. J., Whitehouse, P. J., DeKosky, S. T., Cummings, J. L. Practice Parameter: Management of dementia (an evidence-based review): Report of the Quality Standards Subcommittee of the American Academy of Neurology. *Neurology* 56, no. 9 (May 8, 2001): 1154–1166.

Duncan, S., and Allen, K. Service animals and their roles in enhancing independence, quality of life, and employment for people with disabilities. In A. Fine, ed., *The Handbook on Animal Assisted Therapy.* San Diego, Calif.: Academic Press, 2000, pp. 303–323.

Eddy, J., Hart, L. A., and Boltz, R. P. The effects of service dogs on social acknowledgments of people in wheelchairs. *Journal of Psychology* 122 (1988): 39–45.

Endenburg, N., and Baarda, B. The role of pets in enhancing human well-being: Effects on child development. *The Waltham Book of Human-Animal Interactions: Benefits and Responsibilities*, 1996.

Federal Interagency Forum on Aging-Related Statistics. *Older Americans 2000: Key Indicators of Well-Being*. Washington, D.C.: U.S. Government Printing Office, August 2000.

Fine, A. Animals and therapists: Incorporating animals in outpatient psychotherapy. In A. Fine, ed., *The Handbook on Animal Assisted Therapy*. San Diego, Calif.: Academic Press, 2000, pp. 179–211.

Fitzpatrick, J. C., and Tebay, J. M. Hippotherapy and therapeutic riding: An international review. In C. Wilson and D. Turner, eds., *Companion Animals in Human Health*. Thousand Oaks, Calif.: Sage Publications, 1998, pp. 41–58.

Forbes, D. A. Strategies for managing behavioral symptomatology associated with dementia of the Alzheimer type: A systematic overview. *Canadian Journal of Nursing Research* 30, no. 2 (Summer 1998): 67–86.

Freedland, K. E., Lustman, P. J., and Carney, R. M. Underdiagnosis of depression in patients with coronary artery disease: The role of nonspecific symptoms. *International Journal of Psychiatric Medicine* 22, no. 3 (1992): 221–229.

Friedmann, E. The animal-human bond: Health and wellness. In A. Fine, ed., *The Handbook on Animal Assisted Therapy*. San Diego, Calif.: Academic Press, 2000, pp. 41–58.

———. The role of pets in enhancing human well-being: Physiological effects. In I. Robinson, ed., *Waltham Book of Human-Animal Interactions*. Oxford: Pergamon, 1995.

Friedmann, E., Katcher, A. H., Eaton, M., and Berger, B. Pet ownership and psychological status. In R. Anderson, B. Hart, and L. Hart, eds., *The Pet Connection*. Minneapolis, Minn.: University of Minnesota Press, 1984, pp. 300–308.

Friedmann, E., Katcher, A. H., Lynch, J. J., and Thomas, S. A. Animal companions and one year survival of patients after discharge from a coronary care unit. *Public Health Reports* 95 (1980): 307–312.

Friedmann, E., Katcher, A. H., Thomas, S. A., Lynch, J. J., and Messent, P. R. Social interaction and blood pressure: The influence of animal companions. *Journal of Nervous and Mental Disease* 171 (1983): 461–465.

Friedmann, E., Locker, B. Z., and Lockwood, R. Perceptions of animals and cardiovascular responses during verbalization with an animal present. *Anthrozoos* 6 (1993): 115–134.

Fritz, C. L., Farver, T. B., Hart, L. A., and Kass, P. H. Companion animals and the psychological health of Alzheimer patients' caregivers. *Physchol Rep Apr* 78, no. 2 (1996): 467–481.

Fritz, C. L., Farver, T. B., Kass, P. H., and Hart, L. A. Association with companion animals and the expression of non-cognitive symptoms in Alzheimer's patients. *Journal of Nervous and Mental Disease* 183, no. 7 (1995): 459–463.

Garrity, T. F., Stallones, L., Marx, M. B., and Johnson, T. P. Pet ownership and attachment as supportive factors in the health of the elderly. *Anthrozoos* 3 (1989): 35–44.

Gislason, I. L., Swanson, J., Martinez, E. S., Quiroga, S. S., and Castillo, R. The human-animal bond in children with Attention Deficit Disorder. In R. Anderson, B. Hart, and L. Hart, eds., *The Pet Connection.* Minneapolis, Minn.: University of Minnesota Press, 1984, pp. 105–110.

Hansen, K. M., Messinger, C. J., Baun, M., and Megel, M. Companion animals alleviating distress in children. *Anthrozoos* 12, no. 3 (1999): 142–148.

Hart, L. A. Psychological benefits of animal companionship. In A. Fine, ed., *The Handbook on Animal Assisted Therapy.* San Diego, Calif.: Academic Press, 2000, pp. 59–78.

———. The role of pets in enhancing human well-being: Effects for older people. *The Waltham Book of Human-Animal Interactions: Benefits and Responsibilities,* 1996.

Hart, L. A., Hart, B. L., and Bergin, B. Socializing effects of service dogs for people with disabilities. *Anthrozoos* 1 (1987): 41–44.

Heine, B. Introduction to hippotherapy. *NARHA Strides Magazine* 3 (1997): 2.

Hendy, H. M. Effects of pets on the sociability and health activities of nursing home residents. In R. Anderson, B. Hart, and L. Hart, eds., *The Pet Connection.* Minneapolis, Minn.: University of Minnesota Press, 1984, pp. 430–437.

Hines, L., and Fredrickson, M. Perspectives on animal-assisted activities and therapy. In C. Wilson and D. Turner, eds., *Companion Animals in Human Health.* Thousand Oaks, Calif.: Sage Publications, 1998, pp. 28–39.

Jessen, J., Cardiello, F., and Baun, M. Avian companionship in alleviation of depression, loneliness, and low morale of older adults in skilled rehabilitation units. *Psychological Reports* 78 (1996): 339–348.

Katcher, A. H. The centaur's lessons: Therapeutic education through care of animals and nature study. In A. Fine, ed., *The Handbook on Animal Assisted Therapy*. San Diego, Calif.: Academic Press, 2000, pp. 153–177.

———. Emotional and cognitive responses to interaction with companion animals. *Journal of the Delta Society* 1 (1984): 34–36.

———. The future of education and research on the animal-human bond and animal assisted therapy. In A. Fine, ed., *The Handbook on Animal Assisted Therapy*. San Diego, Calif.: Academic Press, 2000, pp. 461–471.

Katcher, A. H., Segal, H., and Beck, A. Contemplation of an aquarium for the reduction of anxiety. In R. Anderson, B. Hart, and L. Hart, eds., *The Pet Connection*. Minneapolis, Minn.: University of Minnesota Press, 1984, pp. 171–178.

Kaye, D. M. Animal affection and student behavior. In R. Anderson, B. Hart, and L. Hart, eds., *The Pet Connection*. Minneapolis, Minn.: University of Minnesota Press, 1984, pp. 101–103.

Keil, C. P. Loneliness, stress, and human-animal attachment among older adults. In C. Wilson and D. Turner, eds., *Companion Animals in Human Health*. Thousand Oaks, Calif.: Sage Publications, 1998, pp. 123–134.

Kellert, S. R. Attitudes toward animals: Age-related development among children. In R. Anderson, B. Hart, and L. Hart, eds., *The Pet Connection*. Minneapolis, Minn.: University of Minnesota Press, 1984, pp. 76–87.

Kidd, A. H., and Kidd, R. M. Children's attitudes toward their pets. *Psychological Reports* 57 (1985): 15–31.

———. Factors in children's attitudes toward their pets. *Psychological Reports* 66 (1990): 903–910.

———. Reactions of infants and toddlers to live and toy animals. *Psychological Reports* 61 (1987): 455–464.

———. Social and environmental influences on children's attitudes toward pets. *Psychological Reports* 67 (1990): 807–818.

Koenig, H. G. Depression in older patients with congestive heart failure. *General Hospital Psychiatry* 20, no. 1 (Jan. 1998): 29–43.

Kongable, L., Buckwalter, K. C., and Stolley, J. The effects of pet therapy on the social behavior of adults with Alzheimer's disease. *Archives of Psychiatric Nursing* 3, no. 4 (1989): 191–198.

——. Pet therapy for Alzheimer's patients: A survey. *Journal of Long Term Care Administration* 18, no. 3 (1990): 17–21.

Lynch, J. J., and McCarthy, J. F. Social responding dogs: Heart rate changes to a person. *Psychophysiology* 5, no. 4 (1969): 389–393.

Mallon, G. P. Cow as co-therapist: Utilization of farm animals as therapeutic aids with children in residential treatment. *Child and Adolescent Social Work Journal* 11 (1994): 455–474.

——. Some of our best therapists are dogs. *Child and Youth Care Forum* 94 (1994): 23.

——. Utilization of animals as therapeutic adjuncts with children and youth: A review of the literature. *Child and Youth Care Forum* 21 (1992): 53–67.

Mallon, G. P., Ross, S. B., and Ross, L. Designing and implementing AAT programs in health and mental health organizations. In A. Fine, ed., *The Handbook on Animal Assisted Therapy*. San Diego, Calif.: Academic Press, 2000, pp. 115–127.

McCulloch, M. J. Pets in therapeutic programs for the aged. In R. Anderson, B. Hart, and L. Hart, eds., *The Pet Connection*. Minneapolis, Minn.: University of Minnesota Press, 1984, pp. 387–398.

McDaniel, I. What exactly is "equine facilitated mental health & equine facilitated learning"? *Strides Magazine*, Winter 1998, 14:1.

McNicholas, J., Collis, G. M., Morley, I. E., and Lane, D. R. Social communication through a companion animal: The dog as a social catalyst. In M. Nichelmann, H. K. Wierenga, and S. Braun, eds., *Proceedings of the International Congress on Applied Ethology*. Berlin: Humboldt University, 1993, pp. 368–370.

Melson, G. F. Availability of and involvement with pets by children. *Anthrozoos* 2 (1988): 45–52.

——. Fostering inter-connectedness with animals and nature: The developmental benefits for children. *People, Animals and the Environment* (Fall 1990): 12–17.

——. The role of companion animals in human development. In C. Wilson and D. Turner, eds. *Companion Animals in Human Health*. Thousand Oaks, Calif.: Sage Publications, 1998, pp. 219–236.

Melson, G. F., and Fogel, A. Children's ideas about animal young and their care: A reassessment of gender differences in development and nurturance. *Anthrozoos* 2, no. 4 (1989): 265–273.

——. Parental perceptions of their children's involvement with household pets. *Anthrozoos* 9 (1996): 95–106.

Melson, G. F., Peet, S., and Sparks, C. Children's attachment to their pets: Links to socio-emotional development. *Children's Environments Quarterly* 8 (1991): 55–65.

Melson, G. F., and Schwarz, R. "Pets as Social Supports for Families with Young Children." Paper presented at the annual meeting of the Delta Society, New York, 1994.

Melson, G. F., Schwarz, R., and Beck, A. M. Importance of companion animals in children's lives—implications for veterinary practice. *Journal of the Veterinary Medicine Association* 211, no. 12 (1997): 1512–1518.

Melson, G. F., Windecker-Nelson, B., and Schwarz, R. "Support and Stress in Mothers and Fathers of Young Children." Paper presented at the annual meeting of the American Psychological Association, Chicago, August 1997.

Nagengast, S. L., Baun, M., Megel, M., and Liebowitz, J. M. The effects of the presence of a companion animal on physiological arousal and behavioral distress in children during a physical examination. *Journal of Pediatric Nursing* 12, no. 6 (1997): 323–330.

National Institutes of Health Workshop summary. "The Health Benefits of Pets." NIH Technology Assess Statement Online. September 10–11, 1987, (3).

Netting, F., Wilson, C., and New, J. The human-animal bond: Implications for practice. *Social Work*, 32 (1987): 60–64.

Odendaal, J. S. J., and Meintjes, R. A. A physiological basis for positive human-companion animal interaction. *Mondial d'ethologie.* Lyon, 1999, pp. 234–239.

Okoniewski, L. A comparison of human-human and human-animal relationships. In R. Anderson, B. Hart, and L. Hart, eds., *The Pet Connection.* Minneapolis, Minn.: University of Minnesota Press, 1984, pp. 251–260.

Platts-Mills, T., Vaughan, J., Squillace, S., Woodfolk, J., and Sporik, R. Sensitization, asthma, and a modified Th2 response in children exposed to cat allergen: A population-based cross-sectional study. *The Lancet* 357, no. 9258 (2001): 752–756.

Poresky, R. H. Companion animals and other factors affecting young children's development. *Anthrozoos* 9, no. 4 (1996): 159–68.

———. Sex, childhood pets and young adults' self-concept scores. *Psychological Reports* 80 (1997): 371–377.

Poresky, R. H., and Hendrix, C. Children's pets and adults' self-concepts. *The Journal of Psychology* 122, no. 5 (1988): 463–469.

———. Differential effects of pet presence and pet-bonding on young children. *Psychological Reports* 67 (1990): 51–54.

Poresky, R. H., Hendrix, C., Moiser, J., and Samuelson, M. The companion animal bonding scales: Internal reliability and construct validity. *Psychological Reports* 60 (1987): 743–746.

Raina, P., Waltner-Toews, B., Bonnett, B., Woodward, C., and Abernathy, T. Influence of companion animals on the physical and psychological health of older people. *Journal of American Geriatric Society* 47, no. 3 (1999): 323–329.

Robin, M., and ten Bensel, R. Pets and the socialization of children. *Marriage and Family Review* 8 (1985): 63–78.

Rogers, J., Hart, L. A. The role of pet dogs in casual conversation of elderly adults. *Journal of Social Psychology* 133, no. 3 (1993): 265–277.

Ross, S. B., Vigdor, M. G., Kohnstamm, M., DePaoli, M., Manley, B., and Ross, L. The effects of farm programming with emotionally handicapped children. In R. Anderson, B. Hart, and L. Hart, eds. *The Pet Connection.* Minneapolis, Minn.: University of Minnesota Press, 1984, pp. 120–130.

Schuelke, S. T., Trask, B., Wallace, C., Baun, M., and McCabe, B. Physiological effects of the use of a companion animal dog as a cue to relaxation in diagnosed hypertensives. *The Latham Letter* (Winter 1991/92): 14–17.

Serpell, J. A. Animal companions and human well-being: An historical exploration of the value of human-animal relationships. In A. Fine, ed., *The Handbook on Animal Assisted Therapy.* San Diego, Calif.: Academic Press, 2000, pp. 3–19.

———. Beneficial effects of pet ownership on some aspects of human health. *Journal of the Royal Society of Medicine* 84 (1991): 717–720.

Sherwood, N. E., and Jeffrey, R. W. The behavioral determinants of exercise: Implications for physical activity interventions. *Annual Review of Nutrition* 20 (2000): 21–44.

Siegel, J. M. Companion animals: In sickness and in health. *Journal of Social Issues* 49, no. 1 (1993): 157–167.

———. Stressful life events and use of physician services among the elderly: The moderating role of pet ownership. *Journal of Personality and Social Psychology* 58 (1990): 1081–1086.

Trecroci, D. *Sit! Roll Over! Diagnose Hypoglycemia! Good Dog! Is the pooch pal the best glucose alarm clock we have? Diabetes Interview* 10, no. 3 (2001): 28.

Triebenbacher, S. L. The companion animal within the family system: The manner in which animals enhance life within a home. In A. Fine, ed., *The Handbook on Animal Assisted Therapy*. San Diego, Calif.: Academic Press, 2000, pp. 357–383.

————. Pets as transitional objects: Their role in children's emotional development. *Psychological Reports* 82, no. 1 (1998): 191–200.

————. The relationship between attachment to companion animals and self-esteem. In C. Wilson and D. Turner, eds., *Companion Animals in Human Health*. Thousand Oaks, Calif.: Sage Publications, 1998, pp. 135–148.

Vidovic, V. V., Stectic, V. V., and Bratko, D. Pet ownership, type of pet and socio-emotional development of school children. *Anthrozoos* 12, no. 4 (1999): 211–217.

Zasloff, R. L., and Kidd, A. H. Attachment to feline companions. *Psychological Reports* 74 (1994): 747–752.

————. Loneliness and pet ownership among single women. *Psychological Reports* 75 (1994): 747–752.

ABOUT THE AUTHORS

Dr. Marty Becker is the coauthor of the best-selling books *Chicken Soup for the Pet Lover's Soul* and *Chicken Soup for the Cat & Dog Lover's Soul*. Dr. Becker is also the popular veterinary contributor to ABC TV's *Good Morning America* and is the chief veterinary correspondent for Amazon.com. His weekly newspaper column, *The Bond*, is distributed internationally by Knight-Ridder Tribune to more than 350 newspapers. Dr. Becker is also a contributing editor for *Dog Fancy* and *Cat Fancy*, the world's most popular pet magazines.

Danelle Morton is a Los Angeles–based writer with a distinguished journalism career. She has worked for publications ranging from *The New York Times* to *People* magazine and has served as a foreign correspondent, state capital bureau chief, columnist, and associate bureau chief of *People*'s Los Angeles operation. She is the coauthor of three books.